Rating and Underwriting for Health Plans

Rating and Underwriting for Health Plans

John van Steenwyk

Copyright © 2006 by John van Steenwyk.

Library of Congress Control Number:		2006910184
ISBN 10:	Hardcover	1-4257-4391-9
	Softcover	1-4257-4390-0
ISBN 13:	Hardcover	978-1-4257-4391-8
	Softcover	978-1-4257-4390-1

All rights reserved. No part of this book may be reproduced or transmitted in any form or by any means, electronic or mechanical, including photocopying, recording, or by any information storage and retrieval system, without permission in writing from the copyright owner.

This book was printed in the United States of America.

To order additional copies of this book, contact:
Xlibris Corporation
1-888-795-4274
www.Xlibris.com
Orders@Xlibris.com
37753

Contents

PART I	BACKGROUND NOTES
	A. Rating Methods In Historic Context 11
	B. State Regulation Of Rates 20
	C. Rate Negotiations And Competition 25

PART II	BUDGETING AND RISK
	A. Health Plan Rate Components 31
	B. Capitation Rate Budgeting 33
	C. The Annual Budgeting Process 39
	D. Rate Classes 41
	E. Chance 42
	F. Risk And Budgets 45
	G. Distribution Of Costs Per Person 48
	H. Risk Capacity 51
	I. Employers And Risk 53

PART III	CARRIER RESPONSIBILITIES & RETENTION CHARGES
	A. Carrier Functions 57
	B. Components Of Retention 62

PART IV	MODIFICATIONS TO PER CAPITA BUDGETS
	A. Benefit Options 67
	B. Age / Sex Adjustments 74
	C. Other Demographic Adjustments 83
	D. Industry Factors 85

PART V	MARKET AND COST TRENDS
	A. Inflation And Cost Trending 91
	B. The Underwriting Cycle 96
	C. Summary: Market Intelligence 99

PART VI	EXPERIENCE ANALYSIS
	A. Background 103
	B. Analysis Programs And Software 104
	C. Claims Extracts Or Downloads 105
	D. Utilization Rates And PMPM Costs.................... 108
	E. Coding Systems 110
	F. Data Accuracy 113
	G. Data Maps 114
	H. "IBNR" 115

PART VII	EXPERIENCE RATING
	A. Overview—Choice Of Methods 119
	B. Data Requirements 121
	C. Credibility.. 122
	D. Illustrative Formulas And Worksheets............... 125
	E. Presentation And Feedback 134

PART VIII	PREMIUM RATE DEVELOPMENT
	A. Premium Rates: Market Determinants And Options 139
	B. Premium Rate Mechanics.................................... 141
	C. Data For Premium Rate Development 147
	D. Problems With Premiums 150
	E. Rates For Small Groups.. 155

PART IX	UNDERWRITING
	A. The Underwriting Function 161
	B. Organizational Considerations 165
	C. Underwriting Rules 168
	D. Observations On Small Group Underwriting ... 176
	E. Health Statements And Questionnaires 180
	F. Observations On Non-group Underwriting.... 182

PART X	End Notes 187

To the Reader

This book is a product of our work, over a span of about thirty years, in developing rates for health plans, and advising on their application. It is an expanded and updated edition of the text for our workshops on Health Plan Rating and Underwriting.

This is intended to be a practical guide. We mean it to be useful to those who work for health plans as underwriters and rate setters. We expect that it will also be used by health plan executives and leaders—for whom knowledge of this subject matter is crucial.

A health plan expresses its character in how it approaches and deals with its customers. Principles of fairness and equity come from each health plan's leaders, and are expressed in the market through sound rates and fair underwriting rules. Here we endeavor to explain "how to do it" and, in addition, why—and why this subject requires sustained and focused attention.

John van Steenwyk
Health Economics, Inc.
Spring House, Pennsylvania
Fall, 2006

PART I

BACKGROUND NOTES

A. RATING METHODS IN HISTORIC CONTEXT

B. STATE REGULATION OF RATES

C. RATE NEGOTIATION AND COMPETITION

A. RATING METHODS IN HISTORIC CONTEXT

Rate-setting methods have evolved over the seven-decade history of private health insurance and prepayment in the United States.

The dynamics of this evolution essentially involve a move from generalized rates (community rates) to those which are more specific to the risk, group by group. But this has not been an uninterrupted progression: the HMO Act of 1973 stipulated a community rating basis at a time when group-specific experience rates had become the norm. In turn, HMOs took responsibility for providing services within a budget.

The development of group health insurance in the U.S. occurred in several broad phases. The first, which saw the initial development of voluntary health care prepayment plans, started in the early 1930s and lasted about a decade. The next phase—which started during World War II—involved the development of health insurance as an employee benefit.

The initial Blue Cross plans were "community rated". That is, their rates were the same for all groups and all subscribers with the same benefit program. With the advent of health insurance as an employee benefit, paid for by employers, insurance companies began to enter the market, and they introduced demographically-adjusted and experience-based rates, i.e. those which varied according to the costs—as anticipated or experienced—for each employee group. For larger groups, experience-based rates then came to be the norm. But in 1973, the newly-passed HMO Act re-introduced the concept of community rating, or uniform rates for all.

A full history of HMOs and managed care is beyond the scope of this volume. Our focus here is on rating methods. The early influences of the Federal HMO

Act and of State HMO Acts (which also required community rating) have diminished in recent years, as managed care has matured. Currently, managed care organizations are revisiting—or re-inventing—the rating approaches used by insurance companies decades ago.

We will expand on these observations in this volume.

Meantime, we start with a look at history. This provides a context for understanding the rating methods used by health plans in America.

Prior to the development of Blue Cross plans, in the 1930s, health insurance or prepayment was not available in the United States, except for small numbers of people in limited situations. In 1929, a hospital service prepayment plan, one which became well known, was established by Baylor University Hospital to provide coverage for school teachers in Dallas. A national study, by the Committee on the Costs of Medical Care, conducted in the years 1929-31, recommended the development of prepayment programs, starting with hospital care, and cited the Baylor program as a prototype. Budgeting—prepayment—was seen as the key to making modern health care services available to working people. People could pay in advance, so as to be *entitled* to receive care when needed, without having to worry, then, about the cost.

Hospitals embraced the idea: without regular financing, they were not able to keep up with advances in medicine.

The first city-wide hospital service plans were started, in St. Paul and in Newark, in 1933. Shortly thereafter, in 1934, the Blue Cross symbol began to be used by the hospital service plan in Minnesota, and the American Hospital Association established a Hospital Service Plan Commission (later the Blue Cross Commission) which licensed the Blue Cross symbol and tied it to a set of community-service standards. Blue Cross plans, identified with the symbol and the standards, became known for two essential attributes: they assured access to hospital care (as a service to which members were entitled); and each was, economically, a good deal.

The good reputation of Blue Cross was the underpinning for a rapid development of hospital service plans across the country. By the end of 1937, there were 1.4 million Blue Cross enrollees; by 1940, Blue Cross enrollment had grown to 4.4 million persons. A surge of enrollment occurred in World War II: by the end of 1945, membership totaled almost 20 million persons.

The early growth of prepayment plans—in the 1930s and early 1940—occurred under circumstances much different from those prevailing later. Most importantly, health care coverage was not—at first—an employee benefit, paid for by employers. The "dues", or subscription charges, for the early hospital service plans were paid by employees, and were usually collected by "group leaders", volunteers who handled paperwork for their fellow employees. Employer participation, at first, was limited to allowing the enrollment and collection activity to occur at the workplace.

Under those circumstances, it was important for rates to be simple and uniform, "one rate for all". Only one distinction was usual: different rates for single coverage and for family coverage.

As public service enterprises, sponsored by nonprofit community hospitals, Blue Cross plans pursued the goal of universal coverage. The idea was that the costs of hospital care in an area, or community, would be shared equally, so as to be broadly affordable. An appropriate rate, in that context, was based—very simply—on the average per-capita cost of hospital services in the community.

Early group practice prepayment plans, the immediate predecessors of current HMOs—adopted but modified the same concept. Instead of basing rates on community-wide hospital service costs, the early prepaid plans based rates on budgeted costs for their own members, and for comprehensive services. Although the focus of the rates was different—comprehensive services instead of hospital care only—the essential idea was the same: one rate for all—young or old, sick or well.

During World War II, employer contributions to the cost of health care became more widespread, through an exception to the prevailing rules concerning a "wage freeze". The War Labor Board decided in 1942 that the cost of health care coverage was not considered to be part of wages, which were "frozen". Instead health coverage could be treated as a "fringe benefit". Employers, needing to compete for scarce workers, eagerly signed up to enroll their workers.

In the late 1940s—and after the wartime wage freeze was no longer in effect—the National Labor Relations Board and, subsequently, the U. S. Supreme Court, found that employer contributions to fund "fringe benefits" were, indeed, part of "wages". Thus they could be included in collective bargaining. With that, labor unions added their then-considerable power to propel the enrollment of millions more.

As these developments took place, the first Blue Shield plans were started, with the backing of state medical societies or associations. Also, insurance companies, which had earlier left hospital coverage to Blue Cross, began to solicit group accounts. The competitive edge which insurance companies needed to overcome a late start came in part from their willingness to select risks and to base rates on actual or expected group-specific costs. So Blue Cross plans found themselves faced with strong competition: especially in lower-cost groups, mainly those with younger workers.

Blue Cross plans, as well as the newly-established Blue Shield plans, were stung by this competition. They defended the concept of community rating, mainly on the basis that it was necessary to fulfill an important social goal—making coverage affordable to the broadest possible public. This was not only a matter of competitive advantage: it became a public policy issue. The future of voluntary prepaid health care plans—and their social benefit—was seen as being threatened by insurance companies practicing selective rating. The insurance companies were seen as capturing for themselves the "better" business, leaving Blue Cross and Blue Shield plans with a residual population of higher-risk enrollees, which would lead them inevitably to unaffordable and/or uncompetitive rates.

This was much more than a squabble between business competitors. The debate over community rating vs. experience rating in the 1940s and 1950s was put in focus by the then-current issue of national health insurance. A subject of political debate, then, was whether universal coverage would come about through government financing as in other countries, or whether the initial success of the voluntary health care prepayment "movement" should be encouraged and allowed to run its course. The advocates of a private-market or voluntary approach argued that if the community rating principle were consistently applied, near-universal coverage could be achieved without the intervention of government. Phenomenal growth—up to then—in voluntary coverage was extrapolated to forecast coverage of virtually the entire working population. Under the right circumstances, it would only be a matter of time before almost all working persons and their families would be covered.

But these circumstances were perceived to be fragile. It was foreseen—correctly, as we now know—that if each group's rates were to match its own expenses, and if employers were to be relied upon for voluntary sponsorship of health insurance, large groups of citizens would remain uninsured.

From a public policy perspective, community rating is thus seen as a pooling mechanism: a form of income transfer, wherein employee groups which need relatively less by way of health care services subsidize those who need more. For its implementation, it requires a dominant carrier in each area: one in a position to enroll most of the population.

With the proliferation of insurance company competition, Blue Cross and Blue Shield could not maintain the pooling function of community rating. It became necessary for them to follow suit, and to vary rates for groups, based on demographic factors and on experience. But they had regarded community rating as a principle, and their decisions to abandon it came hard: this acknowledged the success of the "commercial" competitors, signaled a new way of doing business, and dashed hopes for a near-universal voluntary system of prepayment.

Part of the pooling or income-transfer function of the early prepayment plans involved providing coverage for the elderly: the slogan was "once a member, always a member", and younger members subsidized older ones. Medicare, which came into being in the mid-1960s, effectively relieved community-rated plans (Blue Cross, Blue Shield, and the group practice prepayment plans) of the need to provide for subsidization of the costs of care for the elderly. The way became clear to have each group's rates self-supporting, with rates reflective of that group's costs.

RATING AND UNDERWRITING FOR HEALTH PLANS

By the 1970s, virtually all large group health insurance business (except that of the HMO prototypes, like the Kaiser Foundation Health Plan) was handled on the basis of group-specific rating, not community rating.

The rating system which evolved for large groups involved "manual" rates, to set first-year premiums, to be followed—in subsequent contract years—by rates based on experience.

Using group-specific rates, two forms of contracting were prevalent. The first, or original form, was called "non-participating": the carrier assumed all risk, and the enrolled group did not share or participate in any surpluses, if experience were to be favorable. With evidence that carriers were making money—taking in more in premiums than they paid in claims costs—larger employers and benefit sponsors pressed carriers for "participating" policies, those in which carriers agreed to return any surplus funds, after accounting for claims and expenses. These distributions of surplus, called "dividends" or "retroactive rate adjustments", became part of a system in which each group effectively paid its own expenses, and in which carriers assumed minimal risk. In effect, a financial deposit was made with an insurance company, in the form of monthly premiums, which was used to pay claims and expenses, with the provision that, after the end of a policy year, any money left over was to be returned to the group policyholder. Insurers were responsible for paying for care within the stipulated premiums, so they sought to make sure that future costs were generously estimated. The resistance of employers to escalating premiums was blunted by the fact that—if premiums were indeed too high—they would get their money back. After all, the carriers would account for the funds, and would return any surplus.

Insurers took two kinds of risks under this form of contracting. The first was for the adequacy of the "deposit": setting the premium rate high enough to cover costs. If the premiums or deposits were not sufficient, the carrier could not look to the employer for additional money until the next year. This led to the second risk: getting stuck with a loss. A big rate increase could lead to the loss of the group to a competitor. With an ongoing contract, carriers could recoup their losses; but if the contract were canceled, this opportunity would be forfeited.

The next step in evolution, understandably, was self-insurance. Claims records showed that health care costs for larger employed groups did not vary significantly from year to year—but just went up, with the general rise in such costs. The risk pools for such groups were large enough to absorb most random fluctuations in use rates. In response, many employers and labor-management welfare funds came to the conclusion that they could absorb the risk of claims fluctuation. They could also assign the risk of high-cost claims—the main source of variation—to a reinsurer, i.e. hedge their bets on claims fluctuations, and still save money. The remaining challenge of rating—anticipating cost increases—was not seen as much of a problem since, in most cases, the needed forecast is only for a year.

Self insurance also eliminated premium taxes. Such taxes apply to premiums, but not to the financial deposits set up to pay self-insured claims.

The refinement of participating contracts, and the development of self-insurance, created a diminished role for "traditional" insurance companies. Without substantial risk-bearing functions, their institutional uniqueness was called into question, and their functions were compared to those of bankers, handling specialized transactions (and large sums of money). Third party administrators, or TPAs, with lower overhead than insurance companies, came into existence, to provide administrative and claims-payment services rivaling those of the insurance carriers.

The upshot of all this was a situation in which larger employers took over the risk-assumption function of health insurance carriers—and then followed up to reduce transaction costs. All of this was in the context of very rapid development in the number of people covered.

The unsolved problem was the rapid increase in health care costs. Larger employers had lowered the administrative costs of health care coverage, but—in the process—had effectively created a "cost-plus" system. Who was to care how much health care costs? Of course employers cared; it was their money. But what could they do about it?

So the costs of administration and paperwork were well under control—but the main costs—those for health care services—seen as being completely out of control. The passage of Medicare in the mid-1960s set the tone for provider charges: this government's undertaking was to reimburse hospitals for their expenses, and doctors for their "reasonable and customary" charges. Those handling the funds, insurers acting as agents for employers, did not have compelling reasons to care about costs. So the general rule, for a time, was for health care providers to bill what they wished, and for carriers to pay, with few quibbles as to the amounts. Costs soared.

Carriers and employers countered with various cost-containment measures, including fee schedules for professional services, and negotiated rates for some institutional services. But these were small barriers against a tide of rising costs. Something more was needed.

Health Maintenance Organizations (HMOs) were seen as an acceptable national-policy response to the cost crisis. President Nixon's 1971 Health Message called for the development of prepaid health plans, as competition to traditional carriers. The models being followed were the prepaid group practice plans, and the foundations for medical care. Advisors to the President described these as "Health Maintenance Organizations". These prototypes had shown that they used considerably less hospital care while providing all necessary services, including preventive services. They also proved they could purchase services astutely, and live within fixed budgets. The HMO Act of 1973 followed up on Nixon's 1971 pronouncement: it formalized efforts, already begun by the Federal government, in sponsoring innovation and reform in health care prepayment. Grants were given to community organizations to study the feasibility of starting HMOs. Federal loans helped the process of development. Employers (of more than 25 employees) were required by the HMO Act to offer HMO coverage to employees, as an alternative to existing coverage. The essence of the change was to put in place hundreds of new organizations which, by design, would operate on a budget, and not as cost-plus conduits for burgeoning health care costs.

While the concept of "health maintenance", gave the HMO movement its name and some of its political appeal, the keys to successful operation, as pioneered by the early group practice programs, included:

1. The absence of financial barriers to care, which enables early attention to disease;
2. Comprehensive benefits—the payment for care in any setting;
3. Avoidance of excessive hospitalization, through vigilance and prior-authorization activities, and also through the availability of prepaid outpatient services;
4. Close attention to budgeting for all services; and,
5. Contracting with outside providers for favorable prices.

The importance of the switch to HMOs, and managed care, was underlined by a belief that, if health care costs were allowed to climb too high, as a percentage of the gross national product, America would be uncompetitive in the world economy. On the domestic front, concern was expressed for health costs exceeding the ability to pay. Those advocating universal coverage, through a Federal system of financing, recognized the need for health care organizations which would live within budgets.

The HMO Act of 1973—and the State HMO enabling acts which followed it—firmly required community rating. This came at a time when community rating was otherwise becoming outmoded, a relic of history.

Many observers, including this author, declared at the time that the Federal requirements for community rating (and for comprehensive benefits) would make the HMO Act a dead letter, an exercise in futility.

As it turned out though, employers didn't care about rating methods. Understandably, they focused on the bottom line—the level of premiums—not on the particular methodology. HMOs in fact delivered attractive rates and benefits, especially to the larger groups, on which many plans focused their first marketing efforts. The ability of HMOs to rein in the otherwise-excessive use of inpatient hospitalization gave them a unique competitive advantage in most parts of the country.

Also, HMOs secured legislation and Federal rulings which allowed them to creatively adapt the concept of community rating, so that they would not be frozen in the rigidity of unworkable rating practices. The main adaptations were:

(a) *Compositing of Rates,* "in a systematic manner to acknowledge group purchasing practices of the various employers" (from the 1976 amendments to the HMO Act). This allowed variations in rate tiers (converting a 3-tier rate to 2-tier, for example), and permitted modifications in the ratio between the single rate and those for family units, so as to adapt to the rate ratios used by competitors.
(b) *Variable Rating,* i.e. adaptation of the subscriber rates to account-specific contract mix and family size characteristics, i.e. higher rates for groups with a higher portion of family contracts, and those with larger families. This effectively defined the average capitation rate as the community rate. Variable rating was formally sanctioned and encouraged by "Guidelines for Establishing Prepaid Rates for Federally Qualified HMOs Under A Community Rating System", published by the Federal Office of HMOs on May 29, 1979.
(c) *Community Rating by Class,* as permitted by the HMO Act amendments of 1981. This allows HMOs to vary the revenue requirement based on "factors which the health maintenance organization determines predict the differences in the use of health services by the individuals or families in each class." HMOs were thus able to use predictive factors, mainly age and sex, to establish rates for groups: this produces higher rates for groups with higher proportions of older enrollees, and lower rates for younger groups.
(d) *Adjusted Community Rates,* incorporating a form of experience rating, were a feature of 1988 HMO Act amendments. Adjusted Community Rates "fix the rates of payment for the individuals and families of a group on the basis of the organization's revenue requirements for providing services to the group".

In time, the cost-containment methods employed by HMOs became widely adopted. The essential concepts pioneered by prepaid group practice plans and by medical care foundations—including comprehensive coverage, encouraging outpatient services and early treatment—were adopted by HMOs and, in turn, by what we now know as the "managed care industry".

There are many aspects to this evolution but, in terms of the focus of this volume, it can be noted simply that community rating played a part. It was first considered a prerequisite for achieving a social purpose. It clearly identified the social and humanitarian aims of early prepayment plans—allied with hospitals in a crusade to assure access for all. For a time, it created a clear distinction for community-rated plans from the rest of the insurance industry. This distinction helped justify Federal financial support to HMOs, and helped HMOs achieve their own unique regulatory basis in State legislation.

Community rating, and a unique way of operating, also protected early HMOs from employers' efforts to get refunds reflecting favorable experience. In turn, this has provided, in practical terms, a shield behind which it has been possible for health plans to develop ways to add to the charges for their services, to share surpluses with providers, to build health plan reserves, and to use profits to attract investors.

It might also be said that community rating—in its simple or original form—"one rate for all" presented a straightforward, understandable rating method to the HMO innovators who did not have insurance industry backgrounds. In the early days of HMOs, this was important: it relieved those who were developing new organizations and building service networks from having to cope with the technical aspects of rating and underwriting. This had a positive effect in stimulating innovation. It also had some severe consequences, in that many HMO managers, untutored in the actuarial arts, made costly errors.

Health plans today build on a dual background: one part rooted in the traditional insurance industry; another part in the practices associated with community rating. The process of development and innovation is continuing.

B. STATE REGULATION OF RATES

State enabling acts provide for State regulation of insurers and specify the conditions under which insurance organizations operate.

While these laws differ in detail, several facts are universal:

1. *The states are in charge.*
2. *Rate filings govern premium rates.*
3. *Actuaries serve as public officers.*

1. The States Are In Charge.

Each State has an agency (or a Commission, Department, Bureau) that handles the State's regulation of insurance carriers, including health care plans. The head of such an agency is usually appointed by the Governor. Some are elected. Generally they are called Insurance Commissioners. Insurers are chartered or established in accordance with State laws. These contain requirements as to solvency. The laws, and associated regulations, also govern rates charged by insurers.

The essential job of each such agency is to assure that the citizens of the State will not be harmed by relying on insurance carriers.

This is important, since insurance is relied upon to maintain part of the economic order on which all citizens depend. Despite their efforts as regulators, States must regularly deal with carrier insolvencies. When they occur, contracts are not fulfilled: claims are not paid, providers are not reimbursed. States under some circumstances must put up money to cover the shortfalls and pay claims.

States also assess solvent carriers to make up for the losses incurred by those which become defunct.

The technical requirements and laws differ for the various sections of the insurance industry, so State insurance departments usually separate their activities between those focused on casualty insurance (fire, auto, etc.) and on life insurance (personal contingencies). Usually, too, there is a distinction between the health insurance business of multiple-line life insurance carriers and those of the health insurance "specialist" organizations—Blue Cross and Blue Shield plans, HMOs, and other health care carriers.

The laws governing Blue Cross and Blue Shield plans, and Health Maintenance Organizations, are generally referred to as "enabling acts". These acts permit the organizations to operate under specified conditions. A wave of Blue Cross and Blue Shield enabling acts in the 1930s and 1940s was followed, in the 1970s, by those concerning HMOs. For the original Blue plans and for HMOs, these acts modify otherwise-applicable capital requirements to recognize the service guarantees provided by contracting providers. The concept is simple: to the extent that providers are obligated to provide services, regardless of whether they are paid, the otherwise-applicable requirements for solvency can be relaxed.

The fact that States are in charge is underlined by provisions that clearly permit or require State takeovers under certain conditions. There are various stages of State intervention. Generally the first stage is one of intensified supervision, in which frequent reports are required by the State, and State-appointed overseers are installed. The next step is generally referred to as "rehabilitation": the State takes over management and attempts to put a regulated insurer back on its feet. As opportunities permit, States may seek to preserve the availability of coverage by arranging mergers or other business arrangements between financially-troubled carriers and those which are solvent. If a group of covered persons faces an interruption of coverage, the State may arrange the transfer or sale of that "block of business" to another carrier.

When necessary—when an insurer has failed—States are responsible for their liquidation. State-appointed liquidators then have the responsibility of getting what they can for the assets of the failed company. If malfeasance is involved—or suspected—the State may sue to recover assets.

In all events the enterprise of operating an insurance carrier, health plan, or HMO is regarded as one of serving the public. The franchise to operate is awarded by the State. The carrier operates because the State permits it. The State's conditions and rules are important and must be followed.

Insurance regulation is regarded as the responsibility of States, not the Federal government. While the concept of Federal regulation is discussed from time to time, the system of State regulation is generally regarded as working well in protecting the public interest.

An association of regulators—the National Association of Insurance Commissioners, or NAIC, plays an important part in assuring a reasonably-uniform national system. Guidelines, forms, and rules developed or promulgated by the NAIC are widely adopted. For example, standard NAIC Annual Statement Forms are used to report the financial condition of carriers.

2. *Rate Filings Govern Premium Rates.*

All State Insurance Departments expect to be informed in advance of the rates to be charged by carriers, or of the basis for rates: the formulas or factors used in determining charges to policyholders.

Generally, in the case of rates to be charged to the public, or to small groups, the requirement will be for a statement of the specific rates to be charged. For large group coverage, the basis of the rates must be cited, and the experience-rating formula must be disclosed.

An Insurance Commissioner must, as a practical matter, be able to explain—to any interested party—why a particular rate has been charged, and why a rate for any group may differ from that for another. These explanations are called for as responses to inquiries or complaints from subscriber groups, or from competing carriers. In most States, rate filings are public records, open for review by any interested person or organization.

The requirements for disclosure serve several regulatory purposes. The State wants to be assured that the rates charged by any carrier are:

- *adequate*—enough to support the risk. (As a practical matter, this is usually reviewed in the light of the solvency of the carrier, i.e. its ability to bear risk);
- *not excessive*—appropriate for the risk, representing a fair price;
- *non-discriminatory*—not favoring class or category of policyholders at the expense of others.

The latter requirement will be seen as important, and the basis for many regulatory requirements. Carriers are, in the eyes of the States, not chartered to "rob Peter to pay Paul". They exist, unquestionably, to pool risks. But they are emphatically not permitted to act as transfer agents in unfairly directing assets or economic advantages from one class of policyholder to another.

Under any rating system, of course, pooling occurs—the lower costs of some groups balance out the higher costs of others. The regulatory requirements for fairness and equity mean that carriers may not systematically overcharge one class of subscribers (e.g. small groups), in order to give a price break to another (e.g. large groups). In the same way, a carrier must treat all policyholders in a class in the same way.

While their overall requirements are fairly universal, State Insurance Departments differ from one another in the details of how they operate with respect to health plan rate filings. Some require rates to be approved before they can be quoted; others follow the "file and use" approach—the rates must simply be filed before they can be used. Some Insurance Departments actively review the content of rate filings, raising questions or objections as appropriate: others are less active, focusing their attention mainly on situations where questions are raised. Most departments rely heavily on the certifications of actuaries concerning the adequacy and appropriateness of rates.

3. *Actuaries Serve as Public Officers.*

In ways which vary somewhat between States, insurance regulation is built on reliance on actuaries as a type of "public officer". Unless they work for a state, actuaries are not public officials: they work for their employers or clients, the regulated carriers. But the standards they observe, as a profession, support the fact that regulators rely on actuarial statements and certifications.

Actuaries have specialized training and functions relevant to insurance and prepayment. Their professional status is recognized on the basis of membership in the American Academy of Actuaries and/or the Society of Actuaries. Members of the Academy signify this with the initials "M.A.A.A.": Member of the American Academy of Actuaries. A Fellow of the Society of Actuaries, having passed the exams for Fellowship, uses the initials "F.S.A."; while an Associate of the Society, having passed fewer tests, is designated as "A.S.A.". These organizations conduct training programs and administer rigorous examinations for admittance to membership. There are about 13,000 U.S. members of the Society of Actuaries; some 3,500 in its Health Section.

Expectations concerning the regulatory role of actuaries are spelled out in detail, in a series of Actuarial Standards of Practice, adopted by the Actuarial Standards Board. Standards of Practice most usually referred to in connection with health care coverage include:

#5— Incurred Health Claim Liability
#8— Regulatory Filings for Rates and Financial Projections for Health Plans
#12— Concerning Risk Classification
#23— Data Quality

#26— Credibility Procedures Applicable to Accident and Health; Group Term Life, and Property/Casualty Coverages

#26— Compliance with Requirements for Actuarial Certification (Small Employees Benefit Plans).

These standards reflect a consensus of the profession and set a basis of what regulators—and others—can expect of them.

A further important set of standards is contained in Interpretive Opinion 3 of the Actuarial Standards Board, concerning Professional Communications of Actuaries. Among other things, this requires that:

— "The actuary should support the position of the client or employer only to the extent that the actuary is satisfied that the position is professionally supportable, recognizing that honest differences of opinion may exist."
— "The actuary should take "all reasonable steps to ensure that the actuarial material is presented fairly."
— "The actuary's opinion should not be subordinated to the judgment of others."
— "Documentation should be sufficiently complete so that another actuary practicing in the same field could follow the work."

In other words, an actuary is expected to express an independent professional opinion. An actuary is also expected to be accountable, to be able to support the conclusions expressed. A universal standard is the same as in physical science: a qualified practitioner, with the same data and information, should be able to duplicate or replicate the results.

C. RATE NEGOTIATIONS AND COMPETITION

A seeming paradox is presented by the State requirements for rate filings. Health insurance rates are regulated, and carriers must comply with rate filings. But there is often an expectation that—for large groups—rates will be "negotiated". If rates really are fixed, how can they be negotiated? If rates are negotiated, how can they be in accordance with the rate filings? Are the rate filings a sham? Are negotiations useless? Are they even permitted?

The answers lie in a maze of history and usages, which can be clarified—to some extent—through understanding the differences in health insurance "markets" based on the sizes of the groups involved. Although the terminology and size criteria may vary from market to market, there are clear distinctions between very large groups (upwards of 5,000 or 10,000 employees), large groups (generally over 500 or 1000 employees), mid-sized (generally those from 50 employees to 500 or 1000), small groups (generally 20-50 employees), and very small groups (fewer than 20 employees, sometimes less than 15, or 10).

Large groups are usually represented by skilled consultants, mostly paid on a fee basis. These generally have high levels of technical knowledge, work expertly with detailed experience data furnished by the carriers, and generally are at the cutting edge of innovation. Experience-rated contracts are usually expected, though when HMO community rates represented a relative bargain (over the cost of other coverage), the fixed—but lower—rates were accepted. Historically, consultants for large groups have focused on retention—i.e. charges for administration, profit, etc.—and have sought ways to reduce that, by shifting some administrative functions and/or some of the risk from the carrier to the group purchaser or benefit sponsor.

With higher health care costs, and with growing competition, HMOs and other health care plans can expect that large groups, and their professional advisors, will test the boundaries of retention. Arguably, there are lower costs for billing and enrollment, in connection with larger groups. If the carrier's rating formula does not recognize such factors, they are likely to be proposed.

In almost all such situations, health plans can expect, as a matter of routine, that the rates will be questioned or tested and are likely to be challenged. A consultant's job is to make sure that there isn't another option that would be advantageous. In any event, a consulting firm is responsible for advising its clients if alternatives should be considered. That includes changing carriers.

The "bargaining power" of very large groups is considerable. Their presence—or absence—on the roster of a health plan can make a big difference in the per-member cost of health plan overhead; their numbers can affect the bargaining power that the plan has with providers. So there is pressure to listen, respond, and to accommodate, so far as is possible or practical.

In doing so, the main rule that health plans must observe is that of non-discrimination: they cannot be in a position of having given any group an advantage which is not justified, and which will not be available to other, similarly-qualified groups. In terms of retention, this means that any lower expenses of sales and billing can be recognized for larger groups—if these can be measured—but charges which don't relate to the size of the group—say for claims processing functions or network development—must be on the same basis for all. A key to this, for carriers and their underwriting staffs, is the rigorous observance of precedents: an understanding that each provision or condition must also be extended to all other groups which are similarly situated. While observing this essential principle, considerable energy and ingenuity can be devoted to establishing what distinguishing qualities justify an exception or a concession.

It would be inappropriate to say that large group rates are beyond the scope of rate filings. This is not the case. But it *is* true that experience rating can make standard rates practically irrelevant, except for the first year of coverage. The most important part of the rate filing, for large groups, is the experience rating formula. While the formula may be fixed, consultants may suggest variations. They will also review how the formula is applied, will want to test and verify the data used, will want justifications for future cost projections, and can be expected to be alert to interpretations that would favor their clients.

Finally, it is true that Insurance Departments can justifiably consider that larger groups can take care of themselves, and do not need their consumer-protection functions. Indeed a frequent focus of Insurance Department attention is often on whether larger groups are in fact bearing their fair share of costs.

Rates for mid-sized and small groups are more of a focus for State regulators.

Here, employers or benefit plan sponsors are usually represented by brokers, who specialize in this part of the market. They are generally not paid directly for their services by their clients, but receive commissions from carriers. They tend to focus on comparison-shopping, usually referred to as "spreadsheeting": creating side-by-side comparisons of rates and benefit features, together with facts about each plan's provider network.

This makes for an active market: one in which there is strong pressure for each plan to make sure that its rates are "in line"—not so high as to prompt or justify defection of covered groups to competitors, not so low as to give up a significant part of otherwise-available revenue. An important part of the rate-setting process involves access to market intelligence, including the rate filings of competitors.

Brokers for small or mid-size groups can be counted upon, also, to challenge rates, or to represent that the rates for their clients—for one reason or another—should be lower. Many feel that they have to try, especially if their spreadsheets do not lead them to a less-costly competitor.

Such challenges are sometimes taken as what they *seem* to be—*demands* for a lower rate. This has led many unwary managers, inexperienced in the employee-benefit marketplace, to accede too easily, and to inappropriately underprice. More often, an appropriate response is to discuss matters in the context of the rules set out in the rate filing, and with precedents in mind. Would this interpretation apply to another group? Does it make sense? Can it be defended? Does it fit in with the rate filing documentation? Would it be allowed? Would it be questioned?

If there are no rules and principles undergirding a health plan's rating (and if the plan does not really follow its rate filing) one can anticipate that that fact will become known, and that the organization will become very vulnerable to bargaining pressure. If brokers and consultants believe they can get an advantage, they will pursue it: it's their job.

It should be understood that the process of "negotiating" rates is similar in effect to other forms of controlled combat: fencing matches, soccer games, etc. The difference is that the rules aren't formal and written. Instead, the patterns of negotiation tend to have informal boundaries. So experience counts. Those new to the market have to learn from experience, so as to accurately interpret what is going on.

State regulation of rates, while sometimes troublesome (in the sense that a lot of work can be involved) can be seen as being useful—even essential—to health plans.

It can be asserted that the main reason why scores of health plans have failed is through their having wounded themselves through inappropriate pricing.

In turn, it should be emphasized is that in the market for employee benefits, price is always a factor; but it's not the only thing. Very important, in the long run, are non-price considerations: network size and convenience; responsiveness to group needs; service to members; perceptions of quality; and overall money's worth.

PART II

BUDGETING AND RISK

A. HEALTH PLAN RATE COMPONENTS

B. CAPITATION RATE BUDGETING

C. THE ANNUAL BUDGETING PROCESS

D. RATE CLASSES

E. CHANCE

F. RISK AND BUDGETS

G. DISTRIBUTION OF COSTS BY PERSON

H. RISK CAPACITY

I. EMPLOYERS AND RISK

A. HEALTH PLAN RATE COMPONENTS

In contemporary practice, health plan rates are usually thought of as two separate parts or components:

1. *Capitation rates*, reflecting *per-capita* revenue requirements;
2. *Premiums* or subscription rates, which convert capitation rates to accommodate market practice: as, for example, 2-tier rates, 3-tier rates, a composite, etc.

A capitation rate usually represents an *average* revenue requirement per person per month, either for the entire health plan or for a defined set of enrollees. It reflects the plan's prospective cost for providing a given set of benefits at a given time to a given population.

In practical terms and for budgeting purposes, capitation rates have the following characteristics:

1. They cover a defined group of persons: the entire membership of a health plan or, more usually, major subsets such as all private-market enrollees, all Medicare enrollees, etc.;
2. They relate to an identified span of time or point in time: this enables adjustments for trends to be applied;
3. They *can* cover more than one benefit program, incorporating adjustments to distinguish one benefit program from another.

Capitation rates include the prospective costs of services, and also the costs for plan administrative functions, and for reserve allocations or capital—building.

Similarly, standard premium rates represent averages: they reflect the average contract mix and family size of the group expected to enroll. The process of setting group-specific premium rates is discussed in Part VIII, Premium Rate Development.

Capitation rates and subscriber rates representing overall averages can be adjusted for application to subscriber groups within the enrolled population. For example:

1. A group enrolled in a more costly benefit plan with greater benefits and lower copays can be charged a higher rate; those in a less costly plan, a lower rate than the overall plan average.
2. Using demographic (age/sex) adjustments, or Community Rating by Class, a group consisting of older-than-average persons can be charged higher-than-average per-capita rates, reflecting the relatively higher costs for the health care of older persons; similarly, rates for a younger group can be lower.
3. A group with higher-than-average expenditures can be charged a higher rate, using Adjusted Community Rates or experience-based rates; a lower-cost group can be charged a lower rate.
4. A group can also be charged a premium rate representing its unique contract mix and family size characteristics.

In practical application, a budgeted capitation rate can be subdivided into many group-specific rates. A health plan can have a great many rates in use at any one time: the purpose of adjustments is to make the rates charged equitable and appropriate for each subscriber group affected.

B. CAPITATION RATE BUDGETING

The rate-setting process for any health plan starts with a systematic process of budget development. Periodic reviews are necessary—to assess experience, and to keep up the process of making predictions.

Currently most health plans budget on a per capita basis—an average amount per member per month. Many years ago, most insurers measured experience on a per-contract basis, because they did not know the number of dependents in family contracts, hence did not have a true count of all members or enrollees. But carriers' data systems now identify each member, so it is possible to keep track of costs on a per-capita basis.

Budgeting is often done by rate "class", as discussed in the next Section. The illustration which follows here involves the average cost for the "private market" or "commercial" enrollees: employees of covered groups and their dependents. Medicare and Medicaid enrollees are different—they are demographically different so, in turn, are their basic health care needs.

If the standard or basis for budgeting is the average private-market enrollees, then a rate charged in a specific situation, based on the standard rate, can be modified or adjusted:

1. From the standard set of benefits to the specific plan of benefits;
2. From the standard, which incorporates the composite demographic characteristics of all relevant enrollees, to the demographics of a specific group of enrollees;
3. From the budget period or the "as of" date of the rate determination, to the applicable contract period.

This indicates the outline of a system: (1) all rates can be accounted for in terms of their relationship to the whole or aggregate, and (2) rates for each particular group will be consistent with the overall rate. If this is done correctly, then the aggregate of all rates charged will meet the "essential test": that they equal the health plans' aggregate revenue requirement.

Capitation rates are straightforward expressions of average per-capita costs.

The basis for each component can be documented. How this is done depends largely on the organizational form of the health plan.

For example, primary care physician services may be offered in an affiliated clinic or health center, and a budget for such services might be summarized like this.

Type of Expense	Monthly Amount Per Person
Physician compensation & benefits: 1:1500 enrollees @ $150,000/year	$8.33
Support staff	6.66
Occupancy costs & supplies	5.00
Other expenses	1.84
TOTAL	$21.83

Or, in the format of a fee-for-service budget, essentially the same expense could be expressed as follows.

Services per 1000 Persons per Year	Average Unit Cost	Monthly Amount per Person
3500	$74.85	$21.83

Referral or specialist physician services, handled on a fee-for-service basis, might be tracked and summarized in a format such as the following.

	Services per 1000 Persons per Year	Average Unit Cost	Monthly Amount per Person
Medical Office Visits	1200	$ 80.00	$ 8.00
Institutional Visits	300	100.00	2.50
Immunizations/Injections	2500	24.00	5.00
Allergy Treatment	100	30.00	0.25
Other Treatments/Procedures	300	80.00	2.00
TOTAL			$17.75

An overall budget for a network or IPA, type of health plan, largely consisting of fee-for-service payments, would look something like the array of figures set forth on the next pages.

ILLUSTRATIVE DEVELOPMENT OF AVERAGE PER-CAPITA REVENUE REQUIREMENT (BEFORE COPAYS)

	Utilization/ 1000/YR	UNIT COST	PMPM COST
MEDICAL SERVICES			
Medical Office Visits	3500	$ 70	$ 20.42
Institutional Visits	400	130	4.33
Consultations	250	150	3.13
Immunizations / Injections	4000	20	6.67
Other	400	30	1.00
			$ 35.55
DIAGNOSTIC SERVICES			
Venipuncture	200	$ 5	$ 0.08
Laboratory	6000	20	10.00
Radiology	1500	150	18.75
Other	1600	70	9.33
			$ 38.16
SURGERY & ANAESTHESIA			
Surgery	600	$ 320	$ 16.00
Surgical Anaesthesia			5.00
			$ 21.00
MATERNITY			
Delivery & Related Services	15	$ 1700	$ 2.13
Other Maternity Services	20	200	.33
Maternity—Anaesthesia	10	600	.50
			$ 2.96
OUTPATIENT THERAPIES			
PT / OT	240	$80	1.60
Chiropractic	150	40	.50

RATING AND UNDERWRITING FOR HEALTH PLANS

Speech / Hearing	20	75	.13
Cancer Therapy	50	1250	5.21
ESRD Services	30	500	1.25
Other	50	150	.63
			$ 9.32

EMERGENCY SERVICES

Physician Services	200	$ 300	$ 5.00
Emergency Dept. Services	150	350	4.38
Other Services in ER	400	250	8.33
			$ 17.71

HOSPITAL INPATIENT

	275	$ 1900	$ 43.54

OUTPATIENT FACILITIES

Surgical Facilities	75	$ 1000	$ 6.25
Recovery Room, Etc.	50	300	1.25
Treatment / Cast Room	50	180	0.75
Other	30	600	1.50
			$ 9.75

OTHER

Social Services, Home Health	20	$ 120	$ 0.20
DME, Prosthetics, Orthotics	250	150	3.13
Dispensed Drugs & Supplies	5500	18	8.25
Blood & Administration	5	250	0.10
Ambulance / Transportation	20	750	1.25
Other	65	50	0.27
Miscellaneous			1.00
			$ 14.20

TOTAL ALL SERVICES $192.19

RATING AND UNDERWRITING FOR HEALTH PLANS

A health plan may construct its average per-capita community rate to encompass a number of benefit plans. Two examples illustrate this concept.

Example #1. Of all non-Medicare members covered by a plan, 60% have coverage for durable medical equipment. The cost, for those covered, is $1.50 per member per month. The amount in the overall budget is thus .6 x 1.50 or $0.90 PMPM.

Example #2. Various office visit copays will be used by a plan. The budget would take account of the mix of copay requirements and, possibly, variations in utilization which are correlated with the copayments, so the overall picture might look something like this:

Copay Option	% of Membership	Utilization/Member/Year	Copay
A	5%	4.0	$0.00
B	20%	4.0	10.00
C	40%	3.8	15.00
D	20%	3.7	20.00
E	15%	3.6	25.00
Total / Wtd. Avg.	100%	3.8	$15.55

The average utilization of 3.8 visits per member per year, and the average copayment of $15.55 per visit, are facts which define the health plan's *overall budget* and revenue requirement. In turn, the rates for each plan of benefits are variations on the overall budget. Thus in this case, if the gross value of a visit were $75, office visits on average would be worth 3.8 x ($75-$15.55)/12 or $18.83 PMPM. But the $20 copay option would be worth $16.96 PMPM: 3.7 x ($75-$20)/12 = $16.96 PMPM. The difference between these: $18.83 PMPM minus $16.96 PMPM or $1.87 PMPM, is the value assigned to the $20 copay—in this scheme of things—reflecting that value as a variation from the standard or average.

C. THE ANNUAL BUDGETING PROCESS

Health plans, as risk-bearing medical service organizations, need good tools of analysis in anticipating or projecting certain cost elements. These involve the analysis of utilization measures, as well as concurrent analysis of demographic and other influences on utilization.

Any prediction rests on the record of past performance and on trends. Trends and developments have to be understood, in light of developments in medical practice and organization.

As part of the analysis process, the demographic basis for health plan utilization rates needs to be kept in mind. Health services utilization is fundamentally related to need (illness, pain, infirmity). In turn this is related to the life cycles of people: the natural cycles of reproduction, growth, maturation, and aging. This makes for predictable differences in the kind and extent of services required by various subgroups within the population.

So health plan management must be alert to year-to-year fluctuations or changes in the characteristics of enrollees; including the possibility of a gradual aging of the enrolled population, producing a general increase in health care needs.

Demographic factors define basic needs. But utilization rates, and hence costs, are influenced by:

1. The health plan's organization—how the physicians are organized, what quality-assurance and utilization review approaches are used, what data systems are used to monitor utilization.
2. The health plan's management—the degree and nature of medical supervision and surveillance, and the control and leadership of other aspects of the enterprise.

3. The health plan's physicians—how these have been selected, and the nature of their training and practice organization. (For example, primary medical practice conducted by family medicine specialists will generally differ somewhat from that of internists and pediatricians.)
4. The health plan's enrollees, in terms of the extent of favorable or adverse selection.
5. Economic and political factors—the costs of hospital services, the levels of reimbursement acceptable to physicians and other providers, and trends in cost.
6. The health plan's location—the overall patterns of practice which prevail in that community.

Finally, as will be discussed further, some health care services, being relatively infrequent, are subject to the laws of chance or probability. No one can really predict the precise number of infrequently-occurring events: and for that reason alone the budgeting mechanism is always an imperfect tool. In turn, it is necessary, in health plan budgeting, to recognize that the budget merely spells out a set of expectations, and that there is an element of risk . . . the expectations may not be met.

D. RATE CLASSES

An overall calculation of the revenue requirement for a health plan essentially represents its budget—expressed on a per capita basis. It can be viewed as an *aggregate of rates* applicable to groups with various demographic characteristics (which can be disaggregated through age/sex adjustments) and for groups with various cost characteristics (which can be disaggregated through experience rating).

The budget can be disaggregated in other ways as well, to produce rates for identifiable rate classes.

The major difference is between Medicare and non-Medicare business.

Non-Medicare business can be further subdivided between Medicaid and commercial—or private market—coverage.

A further division is between larger group business and coverage of smaller groups. As discussed earlier in this volume, these represent different markets, different pricing dynamics. Different utilization rates are likely to be involved, as well. So it can be useful to keep track of these segments separately.

Individual coverage can represent another division, category, or class. In turn, this can be subdivided into categories: employed people, and those who have exercised a conversion privilege.

Another useful distinction can be between early retirees (non-Medicare) and active employees. If accepted for coverage, such early retiree groups often have high proportions of physically-impaired people, with costs higher than would be predicted through the use of age/sex factors.

A further observation on the use of rating classes has to do with health plans which are, in effect, "turning over a new leaf" in terms of underwriting. In such situations, new business, usually accompanied by new benefit plan configurations, may be distinguished from old business.

E. CHANCE

Chance is often thought of as being synonymous with risk: chance and risk are regularly mentioned in the same breath.

It is useful to think of chance as being *an element of risk*: one of the factors that can cause costs to be different from those expected.

Chance can be narrowly defined as statistical variation. It is a natural phenomenon, mathematically quantifiable.

The condition defining chance, in nature, is essentially the number of "exposures". In health care coverage, this is a product of time, the frequency of the events (or services, or conditions) and the number of people.

While it is always true that "anything can happen", the essential concept for insurers is that *there is a definable range of likely variation,* or a range of normal variation.

The rule is: *the range of normal variation is inversely related to the square root of the number of exposures.*

Or, in other words, large variations are to be expected for small groups, less for large ones: more variation is expected for infrequent events, less for those which are more frequent. So frequently-occurring services such as office visits, laboratory tests, and prescriptions are not subject to significant levels of chance variation, especially not for large numbers of people. For such frequently-occurring services, the observed level of utilization for a group of sufficient size, can be thought of as having a cause or a reason, other than chance. (The cause may not be understood or known, but it is not chance.)

On the other hand, an infrequent service, like hospital admissions, is subject to a great deal of chance. Infrequently-occurring conditions, like kidney failure requiring dialysis, or cancer requiring chemotherapy, are likely to have varying rates of incidence.

The familiar example of "pitching pennies" applies. For a few coins, the number of heads and tails is purely random, but for a large number of tosses, the results will be close to an equal number of heads and tails. The more the exposure—the more tosses—the closer the results will come to the ultimate equality of heads and tails.

A more practical example concerns hospital admissions.

If the norm or overall average is measured as 65 admissions per 1000 members per year, or about 275 days per 1000, the range of variation by size of covered group is approximately as follows:

Number of Persons	Expected Range	Expected Admissions per 1000
100	+/-111%	0-137.15
500	+/-50%	32.55-97.50
1,000	+/-35%	42.25-87.75
5,000	+/-16%	54.60-75.40
20,000	+/-8%	59.80-70.20
100,000	+/-4%	61.10-67.60

This means that "good" hospital utilization—say 50 admissions per 1000 versus an expected rate of 75, a variation of one-third, is significant for a very large group. But note that the expected range for a group of 1000 is ± 35%, a variation of about one-third is expected. So such a variation is significant—likely to have an explanation other than chance—only in groups with well over 1000 members.

For a group of 500—a large group for most health plans, it is likely that hospital utilization within 50% to 150% of the expected rate is simply the product of chance.

For visits to physicians the picture is different, reflecting the frequency of such services. Here is an example, around a "standard" of 3500 visits per 1000 members per year.

Number of Persons	Expected Range	Expected Visits per 1000
100	± 15%	2975-4250
500	± 7%	3255-3745
1,000	± 5%	3491-3675
5,000	± 4%	3395-3605
20,000	± 1%	3465-3535

RATING AND UNDERWRITING FOR HEALTH PLANS

As will be discussed further, practical application—assessing whether a group is worse than average or better—depends on a composite for all elements of experience. As will be pointed out, a common rule of thumb is that experience for 1000 employees—sometimes stretched to 1000 members, including dependents—is considered to be fully credible.

The main point here is that there is little real significance in the group-by-group (or doctor-by-doctor) measures of infrequently-occurring services.

In the early days of HMOs, primary physicians were often rewarded financially for lower hospital use rates. Perceptive physicians, recalling their training in statistics, realized that these payments were more likely to reflect chance than any actions of their own. They observed also that hospitalization was not really controlled by them, but by the conditions presented by patients, and by the decisions of specialists. HMOs, coming to understand this, concentrated their incentive payments on measures of quality and service—those which are indeed controlled by primary physicians—and which are not subject to the vagaries of chance.

While much more could be said on this, the essential concepts, in the context of this volume, are that:

- Chance is quantifiable;
- It is a natural part of risk for small groups and for infrequent events;
- It is not a significant factor for frequent events and for large groups;
- It is the main determinant of experience for infrequent events;
- It is also the main determinant of experience for each small group.

F. RISK AND BUDGETS

Part of the preceding discussion concerns a budget-building process—a series of detailed expectations that undergird and justify the rate charged.

But, as we will discuss further, the business of insurance is dealing with risk and uncertainty. It is possible that a budget for health care services will not work out. It is *likely* that it will not work out *exactly*.

In financial terms, risk is defined in terms of a variation from expected costs, or "the extent to which things did not work out as expected".

Health insurance is fundamentally based on pooling. That is, health care costs for a large population can be considered to be reasonably predictable over the course of a year—the usual time span involved in rate-setting. So a health plan exists to pool the health care cost of its members or policyholders—replacing the relative certainty of the larger group for the uncertainty concerning the costs for each person and each constituent group. (This same principle applies to all insurance: the difference is that health services are relatively frequent, compared to, say, fires or floods. So viable underwriting pools for health care risks can be relatively small. Also, the risk changes for health insurance need not be so large.)

So health plans take risks from the shoulders of others. Is their function simply the pooling of risks? Or do they take risks? Both are true. Here are some representative risks which health plans take.

- *New Medical Developments.* A budget, even for a short term, may not take account of new prescription medications or new medical treatments in the process of gaining acceptance and widespread use.
- *New Techniques and Technology.* While some treatment changes can be anticipated through review of medical literature, budget-makers may not be fully aware of what is to come. So surprises can be encountered as new developments are adopted.

- *Provider Network Risk.* The availability of providers to serve members at anticipated levels of reimbursement can involve some risk. Contract negotiations have been known to bring surprises: anticipated levels of compensation may be challenged, negotiations can break down, and there is a risk that unanticipated costs must be absorbed.
- *Enrollment Risk.* Budgets for administrative costs are based on assumptions regarding enrollment volume. If these are not met, the per-capita administrative cost can be higher than anticipated.
- *Market Risk.* A viable market position depends on accurate assessment of the competition, appropriate market strategies, and the use of premium rates which are competitive in the local market. If a health plan is not in step with its market, trouble is around the corner.
- *Demographic Risk.* Demographic changes in large enrolled populations tend to occur gradually, but there is a risk that health plans can (if they are not watching closely) be surprised by unanticipated or unrecognized shifts in the demographic composition of members.
- *Selection Risk.* Pricing and/or marketing of a health plan may result in its enrollment of a substantial number of people with more-than-average health care needs. (The distribution of enrollees by cost level is discussed in the next Section. The processes involved in adverse selection will be discussed later, in connection with underwriting.)
- *Economic Risk.* Unanticipated changes in overall economic conditions may have adverse effects on costs and on enrollment. These may, for example, affect layoffs or hiring in subscriber groups.
- *Health Care Management Risk.* A health plan's budget may rely on the continuation of previous levels of effort and success in case management, and/or on emulating the success of others in arranging care which is both appropriate and cost-effective. But such efforts don't always work, for a variety of reasons, and higher costs may be the result.
- *Regulatory Risk.* Legislative decisions, such as for mandated benefits, can impose new costs on health plans. Similarly, the costs of compliance with reporting requirements may not be fully known when a budget is prepared.

In the foregoing we have not discussed the biggest risk facing health plans—that of inappropriate underpricing. It is assumed that readers of this volume will have this in mind, and will require only a reminder that *this leads the list of health plan risks.*

To say it bluntly, the biggest risk is underpricing. Health plans can survive most risks. This one has fatal effect.

There is always pressure to keep premiums affordable. And, as we will point out, they have to be competitive in the local market. But pressures for lower rates have to be balanced by consideration of risk.

It may be noted that each of the risks mentioned above is manageable—at least theoretically. That is, each of the above risks can be identified, can be anticipated to some degree, and can potentially be minimized. The key to this, of course, is information: a lively and acute awareness of the unique operating environment of the health plan, and the forces at work in the medical and market spheres in which the plan operates.

This in turn leads to the obvious observation that health plan failures cannot only be traced to underpricing, but also to the roots of underpricing: the failure to gather information, and in the failure to understand and recognize risk.

—#—

Finally, it is worth noting that the risks enumerated here are not completely unique to insurance or to managed health care. They are business risks, similar to—though not the same as—those encountered in other pursuits.

G. DISTRIBUTION OF COSTS PER PERSON

Budgets for health care are, as noted, expressed in terms of average costs, per member per month.

This is somewhat misleading in that it seems to represent a regular expenditure, such as for groceries, or the electric bill for a household—varying from month to month but still pretty much the same.

But health care is different. There *is* a regular pattern, but it is one that involves a relatively small proportion of members using a substantial part of services. Health services expenditures are not "regular" for most individuals: they are occasional, sporadic, and sometimes extraordinary.

In all situations a relatively small proportion of members use a substantial part of services. A classic study of physician office visits by the Kaiser Foundation Health Plan, Northwest Region, indicated approximately the following distribution of office visits.

% of Members	No. of Visits per Year	% of Visits
35%	0	0
60%	1-5	75%
5%	6+	25%
100%		100%

That is, 5% of the members accounted for a fourth of all doctor visits.

In terms of total expenses, including hospitalization, the distribution is more extreme. The following distribution is illustrative, and reflects real operating experience.

GROUPING OF MEMBERS BY ANNUAL CLAIMS COST

Category	Percent of Members	Average Claims PMPM	Cost Range PMPM	% of Total Costs
A	15%	$0	$0	0.00%
B	60	30	$1-85	11.04
C	15	200	$86-400	18.41
D	5	500	$401-650	15.34
E	5	1800	$651+	55.21
	100%	$163		100.00%

In this case 15% of the enrollees (Category A) accounted for no cost at all in a year, while 75% (Categories B & C) accounted for about 30% of total costs. Following a familiar pattern, 5% of the members (Category E) accounted for over half of all costs.

The point, in the context of budgets, is that they represent a wide spectrum of people, in terms of health care needs in a month or a year.

In terms of underwriting, as discussed later, the distribution of people underlines the need for efforts to guard against adverse selection.

This can be illustrated in terms of a small variation: if the proportion of members, in the illustration above, requiring no services, were 14% rather than 15%, and if those in Category E were 6%, rather than 5%, then the average monthly per capita costs would not be $163, but rather $181.

As a practical matter, most differences in larger groups are not so stark, nor do they produce such extreme results. But underwriters will want to watch covered groups for "slippage"—do they come to include greater proportions of high-cost enrollees?

A point to be kept in mind, for later discussion, is that there are two determinants for variations in such a pattern of expenses. The first, addressed through the traditional underwriting function, reflects the characteristics of a particular enrolled group: whether or not it contains the usual proportions of individuals by cost level, or more explicitly, whether the group harbors an unusual proportion of high-cost individuals. The other element, of course, is chance or luck.

The difference is that luck is just that. It is transitory: here one year, gone the next. Ongoing characteristics generally have a reason (whether or not known) and persist from year to year.

So budgeting, underwriting, and experience rating depend, to some degree, on understanding these elements, and how they apply in particular situations. In practical terms, does the experience represented by a particular employer, in a year, reflect a pattern inherent to that group of employees—something that is likely to be repeated? Or does it just reflect luck? Or a combination?

On a practical level, health plan managers rely on reinsurance to moderate the adverse effects of luck: if the health plan is responsible only for the first $50,000 or $75,000 of health expenses per person per year, the extreme effects of high cost cases are not so much of a blow or financial shock. Underwriting—in terms of reasonable assurance that the enrolled group is "normal"—is also important.

H. RISK CAPACITY

Although it may seem obvious, risk capacity refers to the ability of an organization to absorb or withstand the variations which arise from risk.

This capacity comes from:

a. Financial reserves;
b. The ability to moderate risk; and,
c. Contractual risk transfers.

Risk capacity also relates, through the above factors, to the subjective capacity—on the parts of owners, directors, managers—to tolerate risk.

Providers often assume some risk. Early Blue Cross plans started out with minimal financial assets: their contractual promises—to provide hospital services—were backed up by contracts with participating hospitals. While the hospitals expected to be paid (and would not have continued as participants if they had not been) they in effect put their assets "on the line"—promising to provide care to Blue Cross members, regardless of payment. This reduced (or eliminated) the formal capital requirements of the early hospitalization plans.

The same is true of HMOs. In fact, the Federal program of grants and loans, intended to stimulate the development of HMOs under the HMO Act of 1973, provided that loans became repayable once an HMO broke even. No particular provision was made for reserve-building because it was apparently expected that provider contracts would minimize the need for reserves.

Indeed they have. Many health plan contracts with providers provide for fixed levels of payment but contain a clause which says, in essence, that the providers are obliged to provide services, for the term of the contract, even if they are not paid. To be sure, a health plan which fails to pay providers cannot expect to find them willing to renew their contracts. But the bedrock protection is there.

While provider contracts give some stability and reduce the *mandatory* requirements for capital, health plans nevertheless—as a practical matter—need the ability to absorb risk and still pay providers. In other words, provider guarantees can't be counted upon for the long haul.

Requirements for capital are contained in State HMO Acts and health plan enabling acts. A national model of "risk-based capital" requirements has been set forth by the National Association of Insurance Commissioners. These requirements define standards which are administered by states in connection with their licensing and regulation of health plans.

Health plans have the ability to *reduce* their risk exposure through:

- Capitation contracts with providers, in which the responsibility to provide care is transferred—in exchange for a fixed monthly capitation fee;
- Reinsurance contracts, in which, for a premium, reinsurers agree to absorb all or part of the costs incurred over a defined annual per capita "threshold" of costs.

As will be discussed in Part III, health plans can *modify* their risk exposure through various efforts in care management.

Further, health plans, along with all organizations in the insurance industry, can *manage* the process of risk-assumption through underwriting—to be discussed further in Part IX of this volume. The underwriting process—to be described further—is essentially one which aims to match the risks underwritten with the rates charged.

I. EMPLOYERS AND RISK

In addressing the needs of health plan purchasers or employers, health plans serve essentially four kinds of functions:

- *They deal with risk*—by absorbing it, by pooling it, and/or by sharing it contractually with provides and reinsurers;
- *They deal with providers*—including the selection of providers and negotiation of provider payment rates;
- *They influence health care*—in specific ways, through prior authorization, case management, etc.;
- *They provide administrative services*—including the collection of premiums, payment of claims, etc.

How much and what kind of each is provided depends on the nature of the plan, the market in which it operates, and the requirements of the employers or benefit plan sponsors.

Large employers have little direct need for risk protection. For them, year-to-year health care costs of covered employees and dependents is reasonably predictable. It is part of a larger corporate budget which includes many elements. While cost increases may be a matter of concern, most employers can anticipate the approximate extent of this.

For larger employers the likely variations in health care costs do not exceed those involved in other business risks, which are routinely absorbed. Smaller employers are in a different situation. Without the stability of large numbers, the possible range of year-to-year cost variations is great.

The "law of large numbers" works for employers—and it works well for those with 1000 or more employees in a covered group. Such larger employers find their year-to-year health care costs to be consistent, with the exception of occasional severe cases, the costs of which can be handled through reinsurance.

For such groups, the odds are that costs won't vary much from a prediction, based on experience, and that any shortfalls are technical ones or failures of knowledge—such as from an unexpected upturn in prescription drug use, an end to favorable prices for hospital services, etc.

It follows from these observations that employers of different sizes will predictably require "products" to suit their conditions and needs.

A small employer is in a position in which—as a practical matter—it *has to* pool its risks with those of others. In effect such an employer must insulate itself from the actual costs incurred by its covered employees and dependents. Without such insulation, a company could suffer greatly from the health care costs of a few people, or even one person. The profits, and the operating capital, of most small enterprises are not large enough to absorb much risk.

A larger employer has a choice. It can "self insure", and retain all or a substantial part of the risk.

This can save money. If an employer perceives that—for one reason or another—its employees require less health care than those in the available risk pools, it will generally prefer to "pay its own way".

This can be accomplished through experience-rated contracts, or through self-insurance arrangements. Both will be discussed further in this volume.

There is a reason why well-informed employers would rationally prefer that health plans retain risk: some risk or all of it.

Simply put, risk enhances motivation.

Employers have come to recognize that the management of an effective health plan involves more than simply paying claims and accounting for money. It requires a great deal of energy, and talent, to manage the finances of health care. Each effective health plan represents substantial investment in information systems, provider contracts, etc. Part of the motivation for creating such systems comes simply from the fact that the organizations are committed—for most of their business—to operate within fixed budgets. Managements are forced to be effective.

So there is a constructive function in health plan risk: it motivates a level of effort which could not be rationally expected in the cost-plus environment which prevailed before the days of HMOs and managed care.

PART III

CARRIER RESPONSIBILITIES & RETENTION CHARGES

A. CARRIER FUNCTIONS

B. COMPONENTS OF RETENTION

A. CARRIER FUNCTIONS

As noted previously, it is useful to think of health insurance carriers in terms of their functions, concerning risk, provider contracting, etc.

The essential ingredients in "managed care" are the functions which have an effect on the organization of services, the choice of providers, quality, and on the volume and the cost of services. These can be seen as distinct from the financial functions of an insurance carrier: collecting premiums and paying claims, etc.

In historic terms, the early models for managed care were the prepaid group practice programs, like the Kaiser Foundation Health Plan, the Health Insurance Plan of Greater New York (HIP), and others. In these, the health plan serves as a financial conduit between the subscriber groups and the contracting medical group or groups. The medical groups are responsible for providing care. In this model, most medical functions are handled within the medical group; the health plan does not have substantial expenses for medical management, network development, provider relations, etc.—nor even for claims payment—and as a result a relatively small portion of total premium is needed for health plan administrative expenses.

The next organizational model, first organized to compete with prepaid group practice programs, is the Individual Practice Association, or IPA. The prototypes for these were originally organized in California, Washington and Oregon to compete with Kaiser and the Group Health Cooperative of Puget Sound, another pioneer in group practice prepayment. In response to the group practice competition, doctors in the affected communities organized "Foundations for Medical Care" and agreed to operating structures which replicated some of the advantages of prepaid group practice medical groups, and also agreed to fee levels which made them financially competitive. As the HMO movement grew, in the 1970s and 1980s, physicians across the country adapted the original "foundation" model, organizing Individual Practice Associations or IPAs for purposes of contracting with HMOs under capitation arrangements.

Because IPAs required a great deal of physician attention to organizational matters, and also because many HMOs prefer to deal directly with physicians, IPAs tended to lose popularity, in favor of the "network" form of HMO organization.

A "network" health plan results from a series of contracts directly between the plan and the providers. An intermediary organization, the IPA, is not involved. The providers are not usually affiliated but constitute a "network" of available providers.

In addition to organizations which are formally designated and organized as HMOs, there are also PPOs or Preferred Provider Organizations.

Some have defined a "pure" PPO as one which does not itself undertake an enrollment or insurance function, but which contracts with carriers for access to its contracted set of providers. This "organization" consists mainly of a set of provider contracts, which stipulate fee-for-service payment rates.

Some PPOs perform an administrative function: that of "repricing" claims. That is, they are involved in the administrative process to the extent of applying their fee schedules, or contractual provider arrangements, to the claims submitted by providers. To incorporate such a step in the claims payment process, the health plan or insurer transfers the claims record to the PPO, electronically, for claim-by-claim pricing.

Other PPO-type offerings are represented by carriers which have contracts with large numbers of providers in their operating areas. In this sense, Blue Cross and Blue Shield plans, operating through provider contracts which stipulate payment rates or reimbursement levels, can be considered to be a form of PPO.

In attempting to classify the medical functions of carriers—as opposed to administrative / financial functions—we can point to these:

1. Health maintenance or "loss control";
2. Care management.

Health maintenance activities, on the part of a health plan, can either be "passive" (inherent in the nature of the program), or "active". Most health plans, by their nature, offer some "passive" contributions to health maintenance. These can be identified as:

- The absence of financial barriers to early sickness consultation (coverage for primary care, no initial deductible);
- Payment for immunizations, checkups, and other preventive services;
- The availability of a "medical home": an active relationship with a primary care practitioner, which improves the chances for early detection and for effective preventive services.

Health plans can also, in varying degrees, involve themselves—and their doctors—with other activities aimed at "health maintenance", including:

- Health education;
- Wellness programs; and,
- Chronic disease identification and intervention.

In the area of care management, health plans can engage in the following:

- Preauthorization;
- Provider selection; and,
- Case management.

Preauthorization is required by many contracts, particularly for hospitalization and for elective surgeries. Services are covered—paid for—if the health plan is notified in advance. Preauthorization can also be required for certain high-cost maintenance drugs, and for other services. The object of preauthorization is to assure that the care is rendered in a cost-effective way, in the most appropriate setting. It can also have a quality-assurance effect or function, in avoiding unnecessary confinements and/or procedures, or in directing patients to providers which have been chosen by the health plan.

Some health plans have come to the conclusion that pre-authorization is unnecessary, or unproductive—in that just about every proposed procedure or confinement is approved. With that observation, pre-authorization requirements are abandoned: seen as unnecessary, and as a non-productive "hassle" for patients and professionals.

This can be interpreted in light of the widespread acceptance of managed care treatment standards. With such acceptance, pre-authorization is seen as obsolete, no longer necessary, since the practices once unique to managed care are now incorporated in generally-observed standards.

Provider selection can be said to have two dimensions: financial and professional. The financial part concerns mainly the agreement, by providers, to the health plan's financial arrangements or fee schedule. In managed care programs, providers agree to accept the health plan's contractual payment (plus a copay if any) as full reimbursement; that is, they agree not to "balance bill", i.e. charge patients the balance of what they would like to be paid.

Selection of providers according to professional criteria, or quality measures, is more complex. Many HMOs require certain providers to be board-certified, and accept that as a measure of quality. All health plans go through a process of "credentialing" providers—essentially verifying that each is appropriately licensed and is objectively qualified.

To the extent that the doctors in a health plan constitute a working community—members of a medical group, participants in an IPA, even members of a hospital's medical staff—an informal process of provider selection is constantly going on. Doctors tend to be known for what they are "good at", while those with less favorable results tend to be bypassed. Primary care doctors assess the results of referrals to various specialists, and the results they see—in treatment acumen, in feedback or information to the primary practitioner, and in patient satisfaction—govern their future referrals.

A further dimension is the selection of practitioners, by a health plan, on objective criteria of excellence. This, so far, has not been done much. One reason for that is that most health plans, for marketing reasons, want to have a broad selection of providers, so they tend to want to increase, not decrease, the number of contracted providers. Secondly, decisions to exclude providers are hard to make, and may have to be defended. Providers who are excluded can allege economic harm, and some have sought refuge in legislation, called "Any Willing Provider" laws. With these in effect, only economic criteria can be applied, and no licensed provider, willing to accept the offered rates of payment, can be excluded from a health plan.

Case management, as practiced by many organizations, involves the carrier or HMO, through its medical staff, taking an active role in following the process of care for a patient. There can be said to be two broad sorts of case management activities: those which apply to chronic diseases, on the one hand, and to short term or acute episodes, on the other.

For chronic conditions, such as diabetes, programs for intervention aim to see that services are timely, that all necessary tests and interventions are provided, and that the patient has access to educational resources which can further self-management. The goal is to help avoid or forestall acute episodes of illness, disability, and the need for more-expensive care. The emphasis tends to be on educating the patient.

The "acute" type of case management, on the other hand, consists of interventions, usually by nurses using telephones, to assure that the appropriate resources for care are known to patients and their families, and are used effectively. Through such interventions, for example, patients may be acquainted with outpatient treatment programs, educational programs, therapeutic resources, and, when appropriate, the availability of hospice care.

A further description of case management takes into account the degree of intervention or engagement: the extent to which it is aggressive: "in your face", as opposed to offering a resource which can be easily rejected or bypassed. While practices are still being defined, a useful distinction involves the process of acceptance of case-management services. In less aggressive programs, a case-management function is offered to patients, and applied if it is accepted. In the more aggressive programs the patient is not asked, and the case management function continues unless it is actively and explicitly rejected by the patient.

As the foregoing review indicates, there is a wide range of health plan activities in the general area of provider selection and care management. Health plans differ to the extent to which they actually carry out these medical management functions. The retentions of plans can vary significantly, to reflect the differences among them, in the nature and extent of their managed care activities.

B. COMPONENTS OF RETENTION

In the nomenclature of group insurance, "retention" is what the carrier keeps—to pay for its own functions, for any applicable premium taxes, to build up its resources, and to pass along as profits to owners. In the usual language used by HMOs, such costs are referred to as "health plan costs" (as opposed to "health services costs") or simply as "administrative expenses", or "administration". A listing of the components of such administrative expenses has been used by Sherlock Company, which surveys health plans to provide an annual "Expense Evaluation Report".

- Sales & Marketing;
- Commissions;
- Advertising & Promotion;
- Enrollment/Membership/Accounting/Bookkeeping;
- Customer Services;
- Medical Management;
- Provider Network Management & Services;
- Finance and Accounting;
- Rating and Underwriting;
- Product Development/Market Research/Actuarial;
- Claims & Encounter Recording & Adjudication;
- Information Systems / Operation—Acquisition;
- Computer / Executive;
- Corporate Services;
- Association Dues & Miscellaneous Business Taxes.

Another way of classifying expenses could focus on functional areas, like these:

- Marketing;
- Account and membership administration;
- Medical and provider management;
- Corporate services.

Premium taxes are levied by many states and are a part of retention. Different rates may apply to indemnity insurance carriers and to HMOs.

These taxes generally relate to the risk-bearing function, i.e. insurance. One of the prime reasons for self-insurance, as noted earlier, is the avoidance of premium taxes.

An element of retention can be reinsurance costs: the costs of providing protection, for the health plan, for the effects of adverse claims experience, usually amounts over a "per-patient", or "per case" threshold, such as $100,000 in a year.

Accounting practices vary on this. Some health plans seek to minimize reported overhead expenses, and count this whole amount of reinsurance premiums as a medical expense, reasoning that its purpose is to pay for medical services. The net costs of reinsurance—the portion of the reinsurance premium which is not returned in the form of claims is, we think, an overhead cost. This is the net cost of insurance, part of what it costs the health plan to assume risk.

Part of a health plan's retention is its provision for risk. And there may be an explicit budget line for profit or surplus. For purposes of the present discussion, we will bypass the issues concerning for-profit vs. non-profit status, appropriate investment returns, and the various ways by which capital is raised by health plans. But we do note that:

(a) The assumption of economic risk requires capital and has value;
(b) Provision for capital acquisition (via paying dividends), its use (via interest) or its accumulation (by way of surplus development) are important and necessary components of retention.

That is, risk requires money. And money isn't free. If a health plan issues stock, it will have to pay dividends, or show promise, at least eventually, of doing so. If a plan makes use of borrowed capital, interest must be paid. If a plan aims to generate its own capital, it must fix its rates at levels which will create a surplus.

This is a topic which, curiously, hasn't been discussed a great deal.

In the context of this volume, it is perhaps most relevant to observe that, in the HMO industry, and in health insurance in general, the cost of capital has sometimes been overlooked. This is understandable when health care costs are viewed as relatively stable, budgeted expenses. But this is not entirely so. It can be noted also that lack of attention to capital is justified when the main risk-takers are providers. But as provider guarantees erode, this is no longer true: carriers are on the line, according to their contracts, and need money to back themselves up—at least to the extent of likely fluctuations in health care cost. As the implications of this come to be better understood, one can anticipate that health plans will make their charges for their risk-taking functions more explicit, and, in turn, that employers which can assume more risk will tend to do so.

PART IV

MODIFICATIONS TO PER CAPITA BUDGETS

A. BENEFIT OPTIONS

B. AGE/SEX ADJUSTMENTS

C. OTHER DEMOGRAPHIC ADJUSTMENTS

D. INDUSTRY FACTORS

A. BENEFIT OPTIONS

Benefit Variations

Variations in benefit programs are necessary to meet pricing objectives and market needs. Low-option and high-option plans—and a variety of each—are possible. State HMO laws generally require comprehensive benefits: hospitalization without limits, office visits, consultations, diagnostic tests—all available on the basis of need. But there still can be some significant variations. A plan can—subject to the constraints of State laws—choose whether to cover:

—Prescription drugs;
—Durable medical equipment;
—Prosthetics & appliances;
—Refractions;
—Eyeglasses;
—Hearing aids;
—Alcohol & drug addiction treatment;
—Treatment of infertility;
—Dental benefits.

Copays

Copayments are another consideration. These generally include a charge ($2, $3, $5, $10, $15, $20, $25, $30) per office visit, with additional charges ($25, $50, $75, $100, $150) for emergency room use, sometimes a larger copayment ($200,

$300, $500, $1000) for a hospital admission, or a charge ($100, $150, $200, $500) for each day of hospitalization.

The first effect of copayments is simply to provide an alternate source of revenue: money at the time of service, rather than as a prepayment. Thus, a $10-per-visit copayment, anticipated for 4000 visits per 1000 enrollees per year, can be translated into a premium reduction amounting to $3.33 per person per month ($10 x 4000 ÷ 1000 ÷ 12 = $3.33). (Depending on circumstances, some account might be taken of the extent of anticipated non-collections.)

In addition to the direct reduction in premiums as a result of copayment revenues, some utilization expectations can be modified to account for lower utilization which can result from copays. Making patients "think twice" before requesting services has been shown to produce reductions in the demand for patient-initiated services such as primary care office visits, and for related services such as laboratory tests. This also works on prescription drugs—those which are perceived to be optional. Copays can also be effective in underlining an admonition not to misuse emergency room services. But copays are usually considered to have no effect on hospital admissions or on major surgical procedures: patients usually perceive that they have little choice in these, or at least a monetary variable is not the main thing on their minds.

Price (and the perceived characteristics of the benefit package) can also influence who joins a health plan. Generally, prices which are considered to be (relatively) low can broaden enrollment and reduce so-called adverse selection. If adverse selection is present (as a result of the attraction of a very comprehensive and high-cost program to people with higher-than-usual needs), then part of a possible "antidote" is offering a lower cost benefit plan, with the objective of balancing the enrollment with persons with "normal" or lesser needs.

Costs can also be modified by the addition of supplemental benefits. These include additions to the regular benefit program such as riders to remove a restriction or to extend further benefits. Important supplements are available in optical and dental benefits. Their availability is important to group purchasers.

An illustrative "matrix" of copayments is set forth below. It is applicable to a hypothetical health plan, and states the PMPM cost reduction from a comprehensive program with no copays.

	Assumed Utilization Rates [2]	Copay Amounts / PMPM[1] Amounts		
Service		PLAN A	PLAN B	PLAN C
Hospital Admission	65	$100/$0.54	$100/$0.54	—
Daily Copayment	250	—	—	$100/ $ 2.08
Office Visit	3750 [3]	$ 5/$1.56	$15/$4.45	$ 25/ $ 7.03
Rx Drug	8500	$ 10/$7.08	$15/$10.63	$ 20/ $14.17
Psychiatric	450	$ 15/$0.56	$25/$0.94	$ 25/ $ 0.94
Emergency Room	200	$ 25/$0.42	$50/$0.83	$100/ $ 1.67
Total Copays		$ 10.16	$ 17.39	$ 25.89
Plus Low-Option Utilization Adjustments [4]		—	1.56	3.13
Net Adjustment (PMPM) [1]		$10.16	$18.95	$ 29.02

[1] Per Member Per Month
[2] Rate per 1000/year
[3] Subject to utilization adjustments for $15 and $25 copay; to 3562.5/1000 (95%) for $15 copay; to 3375/1000 (90%) for $25 copay
[4] 5% of office visits @ $100 each for $15 copay, 10% for $25 copay

    A significant challenge is keeping track of all of the benefits a plan may offer. Since employers have their own ideas of what benefits should be provided, it is fairly easy for a plan to find itself with a few standard benefit plans, but with hundreds of possible benefit variations—in terms of different copays, minor benefit additions and exclusions, etc.

    A useful perspective, referred to briefly in Part II and further discussed here, is the view the health plan's overall operating budget as representing a composite of all of the relevant benefit plans—for all private-market enrollees or all enrollees in a rate class—and then value each component in relation to the average. This relates to an account of expenses *after* copayments.

If the average cost reflects the average benefit plan, it is at least theoretically possible to value each benefit plan on that basis—in relation to the average. Some benefit variations, occurring infrequently, or of little economic significance, may be excluded from this process, so that it doesn't become unmanageably complicated.

It is possible to carry out the evaluation process one benefit at a time: referral office visits will serve as an example.

In a hypothetical health plan, the distribution of members by copay amounts is as follows.

PERCENT BY BENEFIT PLAN

Benefit	Percent
Zero copay	5%
$ 5 Copay	10
$10 Copay	45
$15 Copay	15
$25 Copay	25
	100%

Weighted average copay: $13.50
Assumed utilization rate: 1.00 per person per year (1000/1000)
Average cost per service: $100

For this example we assume that the utilization rate is 1000/1000/year or 1.00/person/year. The average cost per visit is determined to be $100. Utilization of this service is not considered to be affected by copays. The PMPM cost for each of the benefit plans can be depicted as follows:

COST BY BENEFIT PLAN

Benefit		PMPM Cost
Zero Copay	1.0 x $100-$ 0 / 12 =	$8.3333
$5 Copay	1.0 x $100-$ 5 / 12 =	$7.9167
$10 Copay	1.0 x $100-$10 / 12 =	$7.5000
$15 Copay	1.0 x $100-$15 / 12 =	$7.0833
$25 Copay	1.0 x $100-$25 / 12 =	$6.2500
$13.50 (Avg. Copay)	1.0 x $100-$13.50/12 =	$7.2083

In terms of budgeting, the average PMPM cost, for the whole plan, is $7.2083 PMPM and the additions or subtractions from the per capita revenue requirements, for each plan of benefits, can be stated as follows, in terms of additions to, or subtractions from, the average cost of $7.2083 PMPM.

Percent	Benefit	PMPM Cost	Variation from Average	
5%	Zero Copay	$8.3333	+$1.1250	(Add)
10	$ 5 Copay	7.9167	+ 0.7084	(Add)
45	$10 Copay	7.5000	+ 0.2917	(Add)
15	$15 Copay	7.0833	- 0.1250	(Subtract)
25	$25 Copay	6.2500	- 0.9583	(Subtract)
100%	$7.15 Copay	$7.2083	$0.0000	

Using much the same procedure, it is possible to catalogue all, or almost all, of the significant differences in benefit programs. The method illustrated above works when it can be assumed that utilization is not influenced by the levels of copayments. Utilization rates, as well as the copay amounts, could be varied in the case of primary care office visits and for prescription drugs, where the evidence shows clearly that utilization is influenced by higher copays.

A practical note should be added here. Should budget numbers be carried to four decimals? Is it important to track the budget effect of each copay? Neither is necessarily true. The point here is to break down the elements, to gain an understanding of what happens to the budget as the benefit plans shift.

Deductibles

Deductibles should be mentioned here: they are offered as an option by many health plans, despite the fact that a governing premise in the HMO "movement" was first-dollar coverage.

Strong opinions have been expressed, though, that first dollar coverage leads to abuse—overuse—of primary care services. Primary care doctors complain that their time is wasted when a patient's small copay "buys" a visit, which may be for a trivial concern. Whether this is a sound basis for changing coverage can be debated. But it is clear that cost pressures call for lower premiums. Deductibles do that.

But perhaps not so much as may be imagined. As noted, about half of the costs, for a typical private-market enrolled group, come from the top 5% or so of the enrollees: those with very high costs.

What happens at the other end of the expense curve if the first $250, or $500, or $1000 were not paid by the health plan but were to be paid by the patient? For 2006, typical values are approximately as follows:

Deductible	Approximate Percent of Total Costs *
$250	10%
$500	16%
$1000	25%

* Not including prescription drugs

Deductible plus Coinsurance

A variation represents two so-called "major medical" approach: the covered person is responsible for a deductible, as above, plus coinsurance, expressed as a percentage of total costs, until an out-of-pocket maximum is reached.

To illustrate: a $500 deductible (which, as noted above, reduces premiums by about 16%), and 20% coinsurance which applies until the out-of-pocket maximum—say $5000—is reached. So within the $5000 maximum, coinsurance can go up to $4500 per person ($5000-$500). Coinsurance of $4500 means that it applies to $22,500 of expenses ($4,500 / .20). In turn, the out-of-pocket maximum applies when total expenses reach $23,000 ($22,500 + $500).

The first $23,000 of expense for all users accounts for about 78% of total expenses, by reference to the same experience that gave us the value of the deductible (10% for $250, 16% for $500, 25% for $1000).

Thus, we can determine that a 20% copayment, on top of a $500 deductible, subject to an (overall) out-of-pocket maximum is worth 12.4% of the total value of services (.20 x 78% minus 16% = 12.4%).

Trending of Values

Values of deductibles, and or out-of-pocket maximums—of the related coinsurance need to be trended for inflation and re-evaluated periodically.

These values are based on frequency distributions, or continuance tables, that show the distribution of enrollees by the level of expenses and the distribution of total expenses. These are based on observations: tabulations of experience data.

Observations from, say, 2005, applied to 2006 and 2007, would take into account inflation. Thus if the cost trend is, for example, 8% per year, the value of the first $500 in expenses in 2005 would be the same or the value of the first

$463 ($500 divided by 1.08) in 2006. Or, stated another way, the value of $500 in 2006 would be the value of $540 ($500 times 1.08) in 2005.

As a practical matter, it is useful to think of such values as being discounted by the trend rate. So, for example, with a starting point in 2006 and an 8% annual trend, the previously-cited value of deductibles would be as follows for 2007 and 2008.

Deductible Amount	Value		
	2006	2007	2008
$250	10.0%	9.3%	8.6%
$500	16.0	14.8	13.7
$1000	25.0	23.1	21.4

B. AGE / SEX ADJUSTMENTS

Studies of health insurance costs have shown that age, sex, contract type, marital status, and basis of enrollment (subscriber or dependent) have an influence on costs. Also, income or educational attainment is a factor. Any of these, or a combination of them can be used for rating purposes. Adjustments for age and gender are most widely used, and will be discussed in this chapter.

As an example, the following graph shows the relative health services costs by age and sex for an HMO. It is from claims data which we have analyzed, and it shows generally-observed patterns, including:

- higher costs for boys than for girls;
- more costs for younger women than for younger men (largely reflecting costs of childbearing);
- greater costs for older men than for older women.

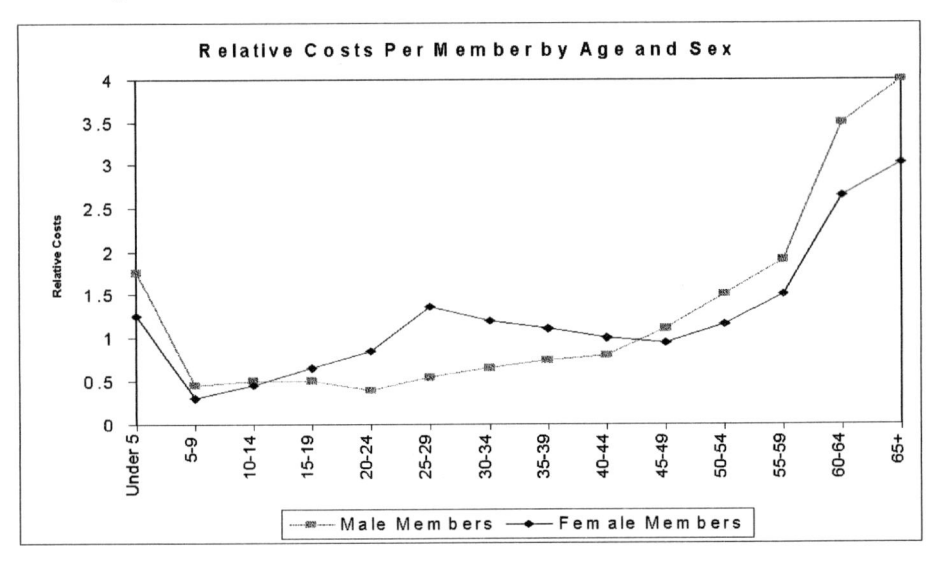

The same overall pattern of relative costs can be observed in just about any population in the developed or industrialized world. The levels of cost will vary, and the shape of the graph will be varied to accommodate the average characteristics of the population described. But the overall pattern persists, as a fact of nature.

Age/sex factors are used by health plans to reflect such population differences. In applying these, a plan must set up standards defining which groups will be affected, and exactly how. (A practical rule is that the demographic adjustments will be applied to any group for which the resulting variation in premiums is at least equal to some threshold, like, say, 3%.)

Theoretically, age/sex factors, applied to a plan's entire membership, will be "revenue neutral", resulting in higher rates for some groups, lower rates for others.

A concern is whether the health plan's contractual costs will actually vary in the way predicted by the age/sex factors. Health plans with uniform per-capita provider contracts face the prospect of modifying revenue through age/sex adjustments, while expenses remain fixed by contract. A remedy, not always immediately available, is to adjust the provider contracts so that reimbursement varies by the same or similar factors. Or the age/sex adjustments can be constructed to apply only to the fee-for-service part of a health plan's total costs.

Will experience actually match the predictions arrived at through age/sex adjustments? There has been debate on this subject, with the point being made that age/sex adjustment factors are—in themselves—not very powerful in explaining variations in utilization and costs. This is true, if the standard of comparison is the costs for a relatively small number of people in a particular year. As discussed in Part II, a group of 500 enrollees (a relatively large group for most health plans) will have, for a year, a predicted chance variation in hospital utilization of about 50%, plus or minus, from a target rate. A group of 1000 (a really large group in most cases) would have a predicted 35% variation . . . just from chance. The degree of variation in overall costs is narrower, but it is still true that chance is the main thing—for a small group in one year. Age/sex factors will prove out over longer time periods—with exposure sufficient to eliminate the effects of chance.

A simple example shows how age/sex adjustments work. Suppose the "standard" group, the entire private-market enrollment of a health plan, consists of just three classes: 25% children, 40% women, and 35% men. Children, in this case, are found to have a cost weight of 0.63, adult women 1.24, and adult men 0.99. The average is 1.00, as follows:

	Percent	Cost Weight
Children	25%	0.63
Women	40%	1.24
Men	35%	0.99
Total/Weighted Average	100%	1.00

A group with different characteristics would have different predicted costs. For example, a group with 35% children would expect about 94.9% of the average or standard costs, as follows:

	Percent	Cost Weight
Children	35%	0.63
Women	34%	1.24
Men	31%	0.99
Total/Weighted Average	100%	0.949

Age/sex factors can be developed by a health plan from its own experience, or, more usually, these are developed by actuarial firms, using data bases which incorporate a number of sets of observed relationships in terms of relative costs. A data base maintained for that purpose would reflect a substantial body of experience, and would show cost and utilization relationships for about 60-100 categories of service.

Such a data base can be applied to the distribution of costs for a particular plan. This composites all of the components of a health plan's cost: the appropriate weights for hospital care, for primary care visits, for lab tests, immunizations, etc. These can be said to reflect the "signature" of each plan's costs. Nevertheless, most sets of age-sex factors look pretty much the same.

Here is a typical set of cost relationships showing the relative overall cost (not including prescription drugs) by member:

	Member Age/Sex Classification	Distribution of Members	Cost Factor
Male	Under 5	4.881%	1.320
	5-9	4.190%	0.331
	10-14	3.774%	0.314
	15-19	3.377%	0.441
	20-24	4.701%	0.366
	25-29	2.714%	0.506
	30-34	4.125%	0.627
	35-39	4.801%	0.687
	40-44	4.640%	1.008
	45-49	3.555%	1.259
	50-54	2.427%	1.717
	55-59	1.757%	2.371
	60-64	1.415%	3.232
	65+	1.064%	3.529
		47.422%	0.955

	Member Age/Sex Classification	Distribution of Members	Cost Factor
Female	Under 5	4.767%	1.191
	5-9	4.199%	0.212
	10-14	3.702%	0.257
	15-19	3.405%	0.569
	20-24	5.586%	0.911
	25-29	4.028%	1.249
	30-34	5.120%	1.202
	35-39	5.941%	1.039
	40-44	5.204%	0.998
	45-49	3.829%	1.276
	50-54	2.511%	1.394
	55-59	1.878%	1.869
	60-64	1.519%	2.388
	65+	1.889%	2.334
		52.578%	1.040
All Members		100.000%	1.000%

It can be observed that the factors underlying the development of the relative cost factors are apt to change from time to time. That is, as the distribution of costs include relatively more or less for, say, hospitalization, for physician services, for drugs, etc., such changes in the overall mix of costs, by category, will change the composite the adjustment factors. So a set of age-sex factors needs to be refreshed from time to time—simply to reflect current conditions.

More urgently, demographic factors need regular adjustment to reflect the demographic distribution of the enrollees. This can be readily done through standardizing the factors. The usual steps in this are:

(1) The factors are applied to the existing membership, and the result is observed. If the average, from applying the factors to the existing membership distribution, is 1.000, then no adjustment is necessary. Otherwise, an adjustment is to be made.
(2) The factors are modified uniformly (i.e., standardized) so that, when adjusted, they produce a result of 1.000. This is accomplished simply by multiplying each factor by the reciprocal of the average factor determined in (1) above.

An example is as follows:

ORIGINAL FACTORS / ORIGINAL DISTRIBUTION

Category	Original Distribution	Original Factors
A	20%	.9000
B	20%	.9500
C	20%	1.0000
D	20%	1.0500
E	20%	1.1000
All	100%	1.0000

ORIGINAL FACTORS / NEW DISTRIBUTION

Category	New Distribution	Original Factors
A	10%	0.9000
B	10%	0.9500
C	25%	1.0000
D	25%	1.0500
E	30%	1.1000
All	100%	1.0275

RESTANDARDIZATION

$$1.0000 / 1.0275 = 0.973236$$

A	.9000 X .0973236 =	0.8759
B	0.9500 X .0973236 =	0.9246
C	1.0000 X .0973236 =	0.9732
D	1.0500 X .0973236 =	1.0219
E	1.1000 X .0973236 =	1.0706

RESTANDARDIZED FACTORS—NEW DISTRIBUTION

	New Distribution	Restandardized Factors
A	10%	0.8759
B	10	0.9246
C	25	0.9732
D	25	1.0219
E	30	1.0706
	100%	1.0000

It should be emphasized that *if the factors do not match the overall population* (that is, if they are not standardized) *they will, in regular use, result in systematically undercharging or overcharging.*

Application of the *per-member* factors to an *existing group* is fairly straightforward. The number or proportion of members in each demographic category is multiplied by the applicable factor, and the weighted average factor is derived.

For a *new* prospective group, the health plan is not likely to know the ages of all covered persons, including dependents. If only the distribution of the employer's *employees* is known (age, sex, contract type), a set of *per-subscriber* factors can be used.

These are built by applying typical age-sex relationships—and pattern of ages and genders of dependents, in relation to those of subscribers—to the per-member cost factors.

DISTRIBUTION OF DEPENDENTS BY AGE & SEX—MALE SUBSCRIBERS

Age Group	Male Dependents Under 20	20-29	Female Dependents Under 20	20-29	30-39	40-49	50-59	60+	TOTAL
20-29	31	—	30%	35%	4%	—	—	—	100%
30-39	34	—	33	6	26	1	—	—	100%
40-49	30	5	32	5	11	17	—	—	100%
50-59	18	16	19	13	1	14	18	1	100%
60+	12	26	14	10	1	2	26	9	100%

Such a matrix reflects data on the general pattern of family composition: women in families are likely to be somewhat younger than their spouses—while some are older; children are generally born to women between ages 15 and 45, etc.

For application of age/sex factors, spreadsheets are used, incorporating cost adjustment factors to enable a one-step adjustment from an employee census to a derivation of an overall adjustment of the capitation rate.

A sample worksheet for such one-step application of age/sex factors is set forth on the next page. On the worksheet the expected numbers of contracts are multiplied by the relevant cost factors and the contract size function. The sum of the accumulated cost factors is divided by the sum of the accumulated contract size factors to produce an index number—a cost (per person) above or below the average.

		FACTORS	
Contract Type	ENTER THE GROUP'S DISTRIBUTION	Cost	Size
Single—Male			
Under 30	17	0.5159	1.0000
30-39	42	0.7407	1.0000
40-49	33	1.0452	1.0000
50-59	22	1.7288	1.0000
60 +	12	2.5766	1.0000
Single—Female			
Under 30	44	1.1215	1.0000
30-39	52	1.3191	1.0000
40-49	80	1.3434	1.0000
50-59	37	1.6486	1.0000
60 +	14	2.1612	1.0000
Family—Male			
Under 30	66	2.1293	3.0451
30-39	89	3.0620	3.6425
40-49	66	3.5593	3.5310
50-59	34	3.7372	2.5385
60 +	20	4.5601	2.2279
Family—Female			
Under 30	12	2.5748	3.3126
30-39	23	3.1105	3.6849
40-49	20	4.2270	4.0277
50-59	9	4.3802	3.4924
60 +	2	4.1624	2.5599
Total Contracts Sums of Factors	684	1,547.27	1,473.68

The group's "Age/Sex Factor" is obtained by dividing the sum of the cost column by the sum of the size column: 1547.27/1473.68 = 1.0499

The factor reflects a relative predicted cost: in this case, about 5% over the average.

Where other health plans are offered to a group, the characteristics of those to be enrolled in one plan or another is not entirely predictable. It can be surmised that a plan's enrollees will match the characteristics of a given group of employees—but this expectation may not match reality: the plan may, for one reason or another (predictable or not) appeal to a subset of any given group.

A technique, discussed (in another connection) in Part VIII (Premium Rate Development) is "backing in" to the demographically-adjusted capitation rate through the use of weighted averages. Thus in an initial enrollment, the health plan's standard rate may be given 75% credibility, with 25% weight to a rate based on the special characteristics of the people expected to enroll in a particular group. Or 50% credibility might be given to a rate based on the characteristics of the particular group's actual enrollees, 25% to a rate based on employee characteristics in similar groups (like school districts, banks, etc.), and 25% to the community standard. Progressively, the characteristics of the particular group can be recognized—given more credibility.

If a "backing-in" approach is not used, and full weight is given to a group's overall characteristics, one way to hedge the bet is to let the employer know that the age/sex rates were determined on the basis of the available data (as from the overall employed group), and that adjustments in the prospective rates may be made if the actual enrollment produces an adjusted rate which is more than x% (2%, 3%) different from that which was projected. Apart from such an adjustment (stipulated in advance), age/sex adjusted rates, once established for a contract year, are ordinarily not modified during the year in response to changes arising from additions and terminations within the group.

RATING AND UNDERWRITING FOR HEALTH PLANS

C. OTHER DEMOGRAPHIC ADJUSTMENTS

Beyond age and sex, other population characteristics can be used to forecast health care utilization and costs.

Income levels or education are sometimes used. Numerous studies have established that those with higher levels of education are relatively more likely to recognize the symptoms of disease and to seek care.

As a practical matter most insurers find their enrollees to be relatively homogenous, in terms of education and care-seeking behavior. The major variations in the use of health care services are found to be between those who have completed a high school education, and those who have not. Employee groups consist mostly of people who have at least completed high school.

Area factors, used by some carriers, can recognize the practice styles—heavy on referrals—present in affluent areas with surpluses of physicians.

Sub-groups with clear differences in health utilization patterns include primarily the urban Medicaid populations, and certain immigrant groups. In many low-income urban areas, the lack of availability of office-based doctors has led to a practice of seeking care at hospital emergency rooms. This has persisted, as a behavior or habit, even when health plans covering Medicaid beneficiaries assure access to physicians in private offices or clinics.

Certain immigrant groups, in the process of cultural and language assimilation, have been shown to have lower levels of utilization than for the rest of the population. Partly this relates to language barriers. Partly it relates to care-seeking behavior learned in areas with far fewer doctors that are available in the U.S. In part, also, there may be reliance on other systems of care: those termed "alternative" here but reflecting care systems which are traditional in other societies.

Some differences in utilization rates affect the uninsured. The importance of this difference is likely related to the length of time without coverage. Those temporarily without insurance are not thought to be significantly different, in terms of utilization patterns, from the insured population. But those who go for longer periods without insurance simply cannot afford to pay for doctors visits, prescription drugs, etc., and, understandably, these persons tend to defer care until its urgency cannot be denied. So "pent-up demand" can be a factor.

D. INDUSTRY FACTORS

Insurance companies have long used "industry factors" as a pricing tool. These are usually listed by Standard Industrial Classification (SIC) codes. A new set of codes, the North American Industry Classification System (NAICS) is now in use, replacing the SIC codes. But the latter are still used for such factors. Long and highly-specific lists are common.

Such specificity, used in forming weights for health care rates, tends to convey a false impression of scientific accuracy.

In fact, the lists are more appropriately described as representing insurance-industry practice, not necessarily factors which really reflect utilization studies and which predict relative costs. Most of those in use are copied from others. Studies which establish actual costs by detailed industry classification are rare, and these are only possible for larger carriers, with significant exposure in many industries and occupations.

A representative selection of typical factors may include the following, among many others.

Agriculture		Services	
Farming	1.05	Religious, Charitable, Political &	
Fishing	1.10	Membership Organizations	1.40
Forestry	1.10	Hospitals	1.25
		Hotels & Motels	1.20
Construction		Clinics	1.20
Paperhanging &		Other Health Facilities	1.20
Decorating	1.20	Automobile Services	1.10
Sheet Metal	1.10	Building Services	1.05
Other Construction	1.05	Recording Studios	1.05

Manufacturing		Transportation	
Clothing & Textiles	1.15	Taxicabs	1.20
Chemical & Petroleum		Bus	1.10
Refining	1.10	Trucking	1.05
Alcoholic Beverages	1.10		
Metal Industries	1.10	Wholesale & Retail Trade	
Tobacco	1.05	Bars & Taverns	1.15
Bakery	1.05	Retail Stores	1.10

Mining	
Metal Ore & Coal	1.15
Others	1.10

Such factors *do not* reflect work hazards: the cost of work-related injuries is covered by workers' compensation.

More likely, the main variable is really the demographic composition of the workforce. Thus it can be observed that industries with a high proportion of older workers have higher costs. This could be addressed directly by the application of age-sex factors.

Industry factors may also relate to an underwriting distinction—the "ease of getting a job", or, from the employer's perspective, the "ease of replacement" of employees. For situations in which minimal skills are involved, and high turnover is the norm, employers may not screen prospective employees carefully, the usual screen (fitness for regular work) may not apply, and higher costs may be the result.

Other industry factors—as for hospital employees, etc.—reflect the often-observed propensity of health care workers, especially those who work in clinical environments, to use more care than the average. Also, some workers, with stressful situations, and ready access to mental health professionals, are regularly observed to be heavy users of such services.

Some "industry factors" may simply reflect negative judgments arrived at instinctively by those who compiled the lists: junkyards are out, so are bars.

These observations suggest a skeptical view of industry factors. Nevertheless, there is no doubt that industry factors are important. If competitors use them to adjust rates, a health plan is practically compelled to follow suit, in some manner. In fact, adverse selection can be the result of ignoring industry factors.

In the case of hospital employees, industry factors usually work out; such employees *are* likely to cost more than the average.

But others are open to question. So it does not generally seem appropriate to burden the rating process by using long lists of factors which are adopted from external sources and which may not make sense. A process is suggested by which a health plan can work toward making sure the industry factors it uses are relevant and sound, or at least have no adverse effect.

A first step is to shorten the list of industry classifications to those which are really relevant to the local market addressed by the health plan—perhaps to 5-15 such classifications.

Second, the results of this can be standardized to the expected enrollment of the health plan. That means making sure that the factors, when applied to the plan's enrollment, are revenue-neutral: that they do not have the effect of lowering or raising the rates.

Third, an effort can be made to ascertain the real relative costs of groups in these industrial classifications.

This can be illustrated first in terms of the adaptation of factors from an external source.

Industry	% of Enrollment	External Factor
Health Care	10%	1.20
Banks, Retail	35	0.90
Schools	20	0.95
Manufacturing	10	1.05
All Other	25	1.00
	100%	0.98

It will be seen that the application of these factors would produce an overall weight of 0.98, and, in turn, a rate adjustment of 2.0%. (A real condition like this could explain why revenue or earnings projections were not met.)

Without really changing the factors, or researching the appropriate factors for the health plan, it is a simple step to standardize them, so that the product, when applied to the anticipated distribution of enrollment by industry, is 1.00. In the above case, this can be accomplished by multiplying each factor by 1.00 / .98 or 1.020408, so that—for this enrollment distribution—they are as follows:

Industry	% of Enrollment	Standardized External Factor (Rounded)
Health Care	10%	1.22
Banks, Retail	35	0.92
Schools	20	0.97
Manufacturing	10	1.07
All Other	25	1.02
	100%	1.00

As internal factors are developed, these can be gradually incorporated.

For example, a set of internal factors, from observed experience, could be given 50% weight (for example) and used to develop "new factors" like this:

Industry	% of Enrollment	Standardized External Factor (50%)	Standardized Internal Factor (50%)	Composite "New Factors" (100%)
Health Care	10%	1.22	1.11	1.165
Banks, Retail	35	0.92	.98	.950
Schools	20	0.97	1.01	.990
Manufacturing	10	1.07	1.04	1.055
All Other	25	1.02	.96	.990
	100%	1.00	1.00	1.000

With a limited number of industry classifications, it is feasible to keep track of experience, and to assess whether the differences in cost by industry can be considered to be predictive. While it is, as suggested, a practical necessity to be aware of industry factors used by other carriers in the local market, it is also important to see that industry factors are applied in a way that does no harm.

PART V

MARKET AND COST TRENDS

A. INFLATION AND COST TRENDING

B. THE UNDERWRITING CYCLE

C. SUMMARY: MARKET INTELLIGENCE

A. Inflation and Cost Trending

As everyone knows, health care costs are increasing, rapidly. This is a big public problem. There are many reasons for this, but three can be highlighted. First, inflation continues in the overall economy. Second, the growing scientific base of medicine indicates that the costs of medical services will increase along with the capabilities of medical science. Third, it can be observed that the costs of personal services, like health care and educational services, tend to rise faster than the overall rate of inflation.

Our focus here is simply keeping up with it: making sure that premiums at least keep pace with costs.

In doing so, health plans keep track of cost trends and utilization trends.

Sometimes these are combined, for convenience, but two distinct sets of factors are involved.

Utilization rates can change over time, and some of these changes can be anticipated. In recent years, there has been a steady rise in the use of prescription medications, fueled in part by new drugs, in part by direct-to-consumer advertising. (For Medicare beneficiaries, Part D coverage has increased effective demand.) Hospital use rates, once on the decrease, are now rebounding in some areas. Various factors, including improved billing procedures, propel increased hospital outpatient costs.

Price or cost trends also must be considered. Inflation affects costs at various rates. Hospital costs may rise at one rate, the cost of drugs at another, and health plan overhead costs at yet another. The value of copayments meantime will remain constant. The effect of these is a blend of the rates applicable to each health plan.

In the context of overall rates (the composite of all the trends affecting each component), it is necessary to "trend" them forward, *from* the time for which they were determined, *to* the time in which they are to be applied.

For example, a rate standard may be developed in accordance with a budget for a calendar year (2006). A rate for a one-year contract effective from April 1, 2006 until March 31, 2007, will have to incorporate 9 months (three quarters) of 2006 costs, and 3 months (one quarter) of 2007 costs. There are various ways to recognize this: the important thing is to reflect the anticipated cost trend in some manner.

Rate trending is always appropriate, even when prices paid by the health plan are fixed for a time by contracts with providers. An underlying upward trend in costs is best met in the context of a regular upward progression of rates.

Group health insurance contracts with employers are usually for one-year terms, starting whenever the contract begins or renews (usually the first of a month), and extending forward for a year.

This one-year rule doesn't necessarily apply, however, to contracts with individuals, people with conversion coverage, and, sometimes, small groups. In such cases, the plan raises the rates on a fixed date (such as January 1) specified in the contract, or without a specified date, when it needs to (and is permitted to, by the State Insurance Department).

In dealing with trended annual rates for larger groups, some plans develop standard rates which change month by month; others develop rates which change quarterly. Rates thus developed are applicable to all contracts entered into or renewed at any time during the month or quarter.

An example of one rate-trending approach is set forth below. It involves quarterly changes in the rate and is based on a $200 per capita rate (appropriate for the calendar year 2006, and centered at July 1, 2006), and an overall inflation rate of 8% per year. The quarterly inflation factor thus is the fourth root of 1.08. The fourth root compounds to the desired annual rate in the case of quarterly rates; for monthly adjustments, the twelfth root is used. (To get a fourth root on a pocket calculator, the square root is simply applied twice. The root function on multi-functional calculators is the xy button.)

One approach is to spread the rate into quarterly components, then base the rate on an average which produces rates that apply to annual contracts—for the quarter in which the contract starts and for the next three quarters.

Distribution of 2006 Calendar Year
Average Revenue Requirement by Quarter
And Development of 4-Quarter Averages

Revenue Requirement: $200.00 (centered at July 1, 2006)
Quarterly Inflation Factor: 1.01942655 (adjustment at 8% per year)

Year	Quarter	Rate	4-Quarter Average
2006	1	$194.32	$200.05
	2	198.09	203.94
	3	201.94	207.90
	4	205.86	211.94
2007	1	209.86	
	2	213.94	
	3	218.10	

The practical starting point for this calculation is the midpoint of the first year—with the $200 Revenue Requirement. This is multiplied or divided by the Quarterly Inflation Factor to get the rate as of April 1 or October 1. ($200 x 1.01942655 = $203.88531; $200/1.01942655 = $196.18873). The quarterly amount is the average of $200 and one of the foregoing: for example ($200 + $196.18873)/2 = $198.09—the second quarter amount. From this point, the quarterly factor is applied to get the other quarterly amounts in the display. The annual rate, in the second column, is simply the average of the rate for the quarter in which the annual contrast is to begin and the three subsequent quarters. These are skewed somewhat by the process of rounding.

A four-quarter average, as illustrated above, is most common. It is also possible to use a five-quarter average. The latter produces a somewhat higher rate, in that it would provide the intended 8% per annum rate boost for a one year contract entered into at any time during the quarter. This overcompensates (and overcharges a bit), in that almost all contracts begin with the first of a month. In most cases, too, the beginning of a quarter is the most frequent occasion for new contracts and contract renewals.

On the other hand, a four-quarter average provides the intended trend only for contracts effective at the beginning of each quarter, and thus can be considered to undershoot the stated trend slightly.

The above procedures can be used to produce listings of trended rates, such as usually required for rate filings.

An alternate approach, somewhat more direct, can be used. That is to simply project to the midpoint of the contract period. For example, if a rate calculation is centered at July 1, 2006, then, for example:

- A rate for the year 2006 (January 1-December 31) will require no adjustment. (The cost calculation is for the year; the midpoint is July 1.)
- A rate for a contract from February 1, 2006, to January 31, 2007, would have a midpoint of August 1, 2006, and the rate would be advanced forward one month from July 1, (or by the twelfth root of the annual trending rate).
- A rate for a contract from April 1, 2006 to March 31, 2007 would have a midpoint of October 1, 2006, be advanced forward by one quarter (or by the fourth root of the annual trending rate).
- A rate for a contract from October 1, 2006 to September 30, 2007 would have a midpoint of April 1, 2007, be advanced by three quarters (or by the fourth root applied three times).

A table of roots follows.

Annual Rate	Per Month	Per Quarter
2.0%	1.00165158	1.00496293
3.0%	1.00246627	1.00741707
4.0%	1.00327374	1.00985341
5.0%	1.00407412	1.01227223
6.0%	1.00486755	1.01467385
7.0%	1.00565415	1.01705853
8.0%	1.00643403	1.01942655
9.0%	1.00720732	1.02177818
10.0%	1.00797414	1.02411369
11.0%	1.00873459	1.02643333
12.0%	1.00948879	1.02873734
13.0%	1.01023684	1.03102598
14.0%	1.01097885	1.03329948
15.0%	1.01171492	1.03555808
16.0%	1.01244514	1.03780199
17.0%	1.01316961	1.04003143
18.0%	1.01388843	1.04224664
19.0%	1.01460169	1.04444780
20.0%	1.01530947	1.04663514
21.0%	1.01601187	1.04880885
22.0%	1.01670896	1.05096913
23.0%	1.01740084	1.05311616
24.0%	1.01808758	1.05525015
25.0%	1.01876927	1.05737126

B. THE UNDERWRITING CYCLE

For many years it has been observed that the financial fortunes of health insurance carriers have waxed and waned in a cyclical manner.

This is called "the underwriting cycle". It seems to work (or have worked) something like this: for periods usually spanning several years, carriers successfully implement rate increases. Competition allows that, because all carriers are doing just about the same thing. The carriers become more profitable and build up surpluses. Then, with larger treasuries, they tend to become more aggressive in looking for new business. In that process, price competition intensifies and rates are "cut to the bone". Underwriting losses result, and surpluses are eroded. Carriers ask providers to hold the line on payment rates. Relations with providers tend to fray. Financial strains worsen. Then, some carriers—generally those in poor financial shape, or those with a strong need to show earnings to investors, or to raise payment rates to providers—conclude that they *must* bring in more money. In turn, they boldly raise rates in advance of the market. This is hard: the higher rates must be "sold". It can be unpleasant, as group accounts resist rate increases. And it involves risk: accounts faced with "out of line" increases can go elsewhere. But, once the ice is broken and this rate increase process starts in an area, other carriers learn of it, are emboldened, and follow suit. Then premiums rise again, surpluses build, and the cycle is repeated.

There is some question as to whether this is obsolete: ancient history, not likely to be repeated. This is probably not the case, even though some of the underlying factors, and the pace or frequency of the cycle, could be in the process of change. Certainly recent history has included periods in which competition has allowed health plans to raise rates markedly (and all did so), and it has included other periods in which competition has compelled zero increases, or very modest and hesitant increases in rates. But in the most recent years (since, say, 2000) there has been consolidation in the industry; fewer health plans and, effectively, less competition.

Volumes can be written about the underwriting cycle. It is a real phenomenon, widely observed, and possibly (according to some scholars) more complex than the description given above. As a practical matter, however, the following can be noted:

1. Health care coverage is highly competitive. Economists would call it a "fungible" service in that, while carriers have distinguishing characteristics, carriers of the same kind (HMO, PPO, indemnity) are essentially like each other. Under these circumstances, price matters ... a lot.
2. For such a fungible service, pricing opportunities depend upon the price behavior of competitors.
3. In turn, this depends on the competitors':

    a. Financial positions; and,
    b. Organizational imperatives.

4. These imperatives, for various carriers at different times, include emphases on:

    a. Growth toward critical mass or market domination; or,
    b. Profits and/or contributions to surplus; and,
    c. Improved payments to providers.

Accordingly, part of the process of rate setting and underwriting involves learning about the rates of the competitors. Spying! Annual surveys circulated among health plans report the anticipated price moves of plans generally. Local information, from brokers or others, may be sought. At the next level, rate strategists can study the financial statements and operating results of relevant competitors, to garner clues as to what they are likely to do. This is relatively easy with local carriers: their Annual Statements and Quarterly Statements make their affairs pretty much an open book. For regional or national organizations, however, it may be impossible to discern anything relevant to the local situation: the regulatory filings may reflect consolidated figures, in which the locally-relevant numbers are simply not visible.

In considering the positions of competing carriers, a useful question is: "What options do they have?" An organization with rising expenses and small or shrinking reserves can be in a position where it will *have to* raise rates aggressively. An organization with a comfortable level of reserves, on the other hand, may be in a position to "see what happens" before increasing the rate of premium rate increases. A carrier with publicly-traded stock will, no doubt, hesitate before bringing on a decline in earnings.

The process of gathering market intelligence—evaluating the competition—can be done to varying degrees of detail.

Market intelligence is regularly compiled by specialized service organizations, which abstract data from Annual Statements and Quarterly Statements filed with States. In most States, these are public documents: it is possible to inspect them and to obtain copies.

Recent history has shown a basic pattern. When available funds permit, health care carriers tend to go slow on rate increases, and can even hold rates in place (if there is a market reason to do so). But when increases are foregone, margins are compressed—mainly because health care costs keep going up. Some plans lose money. Competition limits rate increases. As financial pressures build, health plans are impelled to take the risks involved in implementing rate increases. This tends to loosen the competitive constraints of the market. Thereafter, rate increases tend to conform to the new competitive norm, rates generally increase, carriers build reserves, and the stage is set for another cycle.

Again, it could be that circumstances have changed. Dampening factors are, first, the decline in health plan competition, and second, the increasing prevalence of carriers with publicly-traded stocks. Since stock prices reflect earning prospects, and the latter depend on rates, there is, in such organizations, a strong incentive to keep up the pace of premium increases, and to implement these with a steely resolve.

C. SUMMARY: MARKET INTELLIGENCE

It would be a mistake to conclude, from the technical material on budgeting and trending, that health plan rates come only from the rarified world of actuarial science. They also exist in the world of commerce and competition.

The fact that this competition exists in a regulated environment means that it is possible—in most situations—to keep track of competitors: what they are charging, whether they are growing, their charges in approaches or strategies, their financial positions. State insurance departments, then, are not simply regulators: they are also rich resources of competitive information.

Health plan managers have to be informed about their markets: getting feedback from client groups, from brokers—and from the community of providers whose services constitute the end product of managed care.

There are good reasons for making sure that rates are "in line" with the competition. These concern risk selection. Rates which are "too high" generally tend to invite adverse selection: they are acceptable mainly to groups which have no better alternatives.

PART VI

EXPERIENCE ANALYSIS

A. BACKGROUND

B. ANALYSIS PROGRAMS AND SOFTWARE

C. CLAIMS EXTRACTS OR DOWNLOADS

D. UTILIZATION RATES & PMPM COSTS

E. CODING SYSTEMS

F. DATA ACCURACY

G. DATA MAPS

H. "IBNR"

A. BACKGROUND

An important part of the rate setting job is the evaluation of experience and setting renewal rates for current subscriber groups.

Many in a health plan will have an interest in cost and utilization data: for example, the Medical Director and his/her staff will likely be on the lookout for utilization trends and will be concerned with analyses of provider performance. The finance staff will be alert to cost trends, and will use overall experience data to assemble input to the annual budgeting process. The underwriting staff, for its part, will be especially concerned with group-to-group cost differences, and their explanations.

The following notes concern claims data in general, with an emphasis on information to be used for rate setting.

B. ANALYSIS PROGRAMS AND SOFTWARE

There are several kinds of software programs which are used to summarize and analyze claims data. One kind might be called "system-embedded": the tabulation software that comes with the claims processing system, used to present a series of standard reports. Generally, these will present an overall picture of operations. But more specialized reports are required for various purposes. The "drill-down" capability built into most systems enables staff members to run specific queries, such as "number of members with mammograms" or "total amount paid to Memorial Hospital", or "CPT codes used most frequently by Dr. Jones".

Other programs might be described as "specific-use" programs. An example is the quality assurance reports required under HEDIS (Healthplan Employer Data and Information Set).

A third type—general purpose tabulation and statistical programs—are very flexible in terms of output, and generally operate on personal computers, using data downloaded from a mainframe. Such programs include ACCESS, from Microsoft Corporation, the SAS System, from The SAS Institute in Cary, NC, and SPSS from SPSS Inc. in Chicago. These differ in terms of how "user-friendly" they are, speed, and in their capabilities. But the main point is that such programs allow extensive analyses to be done in special-purpose applications, without burdening the operating system for anything more than a data download.

C. CLAIMS EXTRACTS OR DOWNLOADS

The basic data source is the detailed electronic record of each claim or encounter. These records are kept mostly for administrative purposes; to account for money and services. They are also a rich source of data for analysis. The electronic records used for analysis are often referred to as a "claims extract" since they represent an extract or selection from the descriptive items regarding each claim. They are also referred to as a "download" from the health plan's larger computer file.

Such an extract or download includes only the data needed for analytic purposes: a great deal of information, needed for administrative purposes, can be excluded.

The following is a representative list of data elements in such an extract or download. The "Member Description" data is routinely imported from the membership file, and it is keyed to the member number. The rest of the data comes from the claim or the record of an encounter or service.

CONTENTS OF CLAIMS EXTRACT

Category	Data Element	Note
MEMBER DESCRIPTION	Member number	Plan assigned number
	Year, month, day of birth	YY/MM/DD
	Member gender	M/F
	Group number	Plan assigned number
	PCP number for member	Plan assigned number
SERVICE DESCRIPTION	Count of services	Number shown on invoice
	Service code	CPT, UB, HCPCS
	Date of service / admission date	YY/MM/DD
	Discharge date for hospital stay	YY/MM/DD
	Service location	Standard code
DIAGNOSES	Primary diagnosis	ICD-9
	Secondary diagnosis	ICD-9
PROVIDER	Provider number	Plan assigned number
	Provider code	Plan code
MONEY	Billed amount	$ billed by provider
	Allowed amount	$ allowed by plan
	Copay amount	$ Copay
	COB amount	$ COB
	Paid amount	$ allowed less $ copay & $ COB
	Date invoice received / logged in	YY/MM/DD
	Date invoice paid	YY/MM/DD
	Claims status (pending, denied, paid, etc.)	Plan code

Each line of a claims record can be visualized as representing a billed service, with a full description of what was done, when, for whom, where, by what provider, the amount billed, the amount paid, etc. Where the record is of capitated services, the information on billing does not apply, and the record is not of a claim, but of an encounter or service. Some systems are configured to record and display a dollar value for each capitated encounter, even though no claims were paid.

The key elements, for each service, are the service code, the date of service, and the amount of payment. If reports by age, sex, and eligibility category are to be made, that information is an essential part of the claims record to be used. If claims are to be analyzed by diagnosis, then that information, which is part of most claims, needs to be part of the download or claims tape extract.

D. UTILIZATION RATES AND PMPM COSTS

A typical report on utilization involves, for each identified type of service, three measures:

- Utilization;
- Unit Cost;
- PMPM Costs.

Utilization rates represent the count of services divided by an appropriate denominator. For example, 25,000 hospital days divided by 10 (thousand member-years) would equate to 250 days per 1000 enrollees per year. If the population in question were 1/3 children and 2/3 adults, the resulting rates might be expressed separately for each sub-group, as follows:

Classification	Hospital Days	Thousand/Member Years	Hospital Days/1000/Year
Adults	2,000	6.667	300
Children	500	3.333	150
All	2,500	10.000	250

Similarly, utilization data can be broken down by subscriber group, using the group number to identify the numerator—claims which "belong" to the group in question, and using the group number to compile the membership list and the denominator.

Monthly per member costs (PMPM costs) reflect both the utilization rate for the type of service involved and the average unit cost, as shown. The arithmetic relationship can be understood in terms of the following formula:

Utilization Rate (per 1,000/year) x Avg. Unit Cost/12 (months)/1,000 (Persons) equals Monthly Cost per Member

Example: 300 x $1000 / 12 / 1,000 = $25.00.

Dividing by 12 and by 1000 (or by 12,000) reconciles the two common methods of reporting: *utilization* on the basis of *1,000 eligibles for a year* and *costs* on a *monthly per capita* basis.

Discussions of utilization, and industry comparisons, are usually in terms of such annual utilization rates. (Alternatively, utilization can be reported on a *monthly* basis, rather than annual; or per person, or per 100 persons rather than per 1,000 persons—but either involve very small or fractional numbers, which are harder to use. Annual rates, per thousand people, do not usually require expression in terms of fractional numbers, and are most widely used.

RATING AND UNDERWRITING FOR HEALTH PLANS

E. CODING SYSTEMS

Well-developed coding systems define and describe medical services: there is a code for just about every possible service, and for all things used in treatment. These are the basis for billing: they also form the backbone of numeric tallies of utilization.

The American Medical Association has sponsored the development of the Code of Procedural Terminology, commonly referred to as "CPT codes", which describe every type of physician service, with detailed descriptions which distinguish one service from another. The CPT codes are updated annually. Each code contains five digits, from 00100 to 99499. Not every number is used: there is room for expansion.

Surgical procedures are organized by anatomical systems: integumentary, orthopedic, etc. Code 10040 describes acne surgery, for example, Code 27550 describes surgical treatment of a knee dislocation. Over 4,000 surgical procedures are described.

In addition to the CPT codes, an extension of the ICD codes (referred to below) describes surgical procedures, and that set of codes is used by certain providers and payers.

CPT codes describe over 2000 radiological services, approximately 1400 laboratory or pathology services, and about 1000 medical exams or procedures.

The E & M (Evaluation and Management) codes, a subset of the CPT codes in the numeric code range over 99,200, provide detail in describing medical care encounters which do not involve procedures. These codes were specifically developed to give expression to desirable physician functions: diagnosis, listening, counseling, evaluating, managing. Two examples can serve for illustration. Code 99201 describes an office or outpatient visit of a new patient requiring "a problem-focused history; a problem-focused examination, and straightforward medical decision making". Code 99202, also for a new patient, describes a situation in which an *expanded* problem-focused history is required. These E & M codes, over 100 of them, describe a range of medical services in various settings, including inpatient care, emergency room services, and office encounters.

To describe medical supplies, devices, and certain services, such as ambulance services, the U. S. Government maintains a set of codes referred to as "HCPCS II". These consist of four digits and a letter. For example, Codes A6216 through A6233 describe various kinds and sizes of gauze dressings.

In addition, to describe hospital inpatient or outpatient services, there are so-called "UB" or Uniform Billing codes. These are 3-digit codes: for example, Code 331 describes a chemotherapy injection; Code 100 describes an inclusive charge for hospitalization (including room and board and ancillary services); Code 421 is for a physical therapy visit.

Hospital confinements—the inpatient services of hospitals—can also be described according to the Diagnosis Related Group, or DRG, methodology. This is a system describing about 500 patient characteristics and sets of needs. For example, hospitalization for uncomplicated childbirth is listed under DRG 373, while that for treatment of a heart attack would be under DRG Codes 121, 122, or 123.

A subset of HCPCS codes is used to describe dental procedures: These number about 600, and consist of a 4-digit code with the letter "D" as a prefix.

Prescription drugs, likewise, are coded according to a numeric system (National Drug Codes, or NDC) which classifies them according to therapeutic category.

In addition, the *reason* for every service, in terms of *diagnosis*, is required in each claim, in the form of a description (numeric with some alphabetic extensions) using the ICD system, the International Classification of Diseases. The edition currently in use is referred to as ICD-9-CM, referring to the 9th revision of the International Classification of Diseases, with Clinical Modification (CM). Clinical modifications were added to this system by the United States National Center for Health Statistics, to make the descriptions more specific.

In addition, the ICD-9 system has been expanded to describe surgical procedures, as mentioned above. This uses a classification system developed by the World Health Organization (WHO).

The 9th revision of the International Classification of Diseases dates back to 1977, but has been periodically updated. In 1993 WHO adopted a system described as ICD-10. It is being used by WHO for statistical tracking, and at some point is likely to come into common use, in this country, essentially replacing ICD-9. There appears to be no urgency—on the domestic front—in implementing the shift to ICD-10. This change has been resisted by carriers and providers, which generally find ICD-9 to be adequate.

#

A basic observation is *there is a code for everything*, and these codes are routinely used in accounting for services rendered and in seeking reimbursement. The code sets are regularly updated to reflect new procedures. So, as a matter of routine, almost every claim or encounter is regularly described in standard codes. In turn, the data for almost any kind of analysis is (or should be) readily available. (The exceptions are when data systems break down, or when input—from providers—is absent or faulty.)

F. DATA ACCURACY

Claims data are rarely "perfect". When providers fill out claims forms, their orientation, generally, is to record enough information to be sure that the claims will be paid. When received by the health plan, claims go through an editing process, and, as a result of that, some claims are returned for additional information. But the editing process is not always complete: for example, it is possible, in many cases, to record an inaccurate diagnosis without disqualifying the claim from payment. Diagnoses for the same person may vary from one provider to another. Health plan or provider administrative errors sometimes are reflected in claims records: for example, an occasional childbirth might be attributed to a man, or a claim might be listed as paid prior to the date of service.

A zero error rate is a goal. But most practical purposes of recording utilization rates and costs is served even if there are small errors. Statistical analyses are generally focused on highlights of claims experience and the data supporting them is almost always found to be robust enough for practical purposes.

G. DATA MAPS

The key to summarizing utilization data is the development of an appropriate "data map" or set of code specifications for producing reports. The "map" specifies the codes which create meaningful aggregates: office visits, x-rays, lab tests, etc.

As an illustration, the codes or code ranges for certain diagnostic services would be listed as follows:

	CPT	HCPCS	UB
Venipuncture	36400-36425	G0001	—
Lab—Multichannel	80002-80092	G0060	303-304
Lab—Chemistry & Toxicology	82000-84999	P2000-P-5000	301
Lab—Hematology	85000-85999	P9010-P9024	305

There are no "standard" data maps: each is developed according to the purposes for which it is made, and the preferences of the users. A consideration is the degree of detail to be incorporated in the report. It may be observed that the preparation of a data map is a lot of work, and that the classifications have to reflect some understanding of the clinical content of the record. It can also be noted that comparative analyses depend on uniformity in the service descriptions, i.e. use of the same map. While it may seem that descriptive terms like "office visits" can be relied upon to describe the same thing in all cases, this is really not the case! Tabulations are the same only when the same data definitions are used.

H. "IBNR"

A record of claims *paid* will not—obviously—be an adequate, or complete, record of claims incurred in a recent period of time. Until *all* the claims are paid—a process which can take a year or more—an estimate of outstanding claims is necessary.

There is usually a time gap—commonly several weeks—between the time a service is performed and the time a bill is received and recorded by a health plan. Another span of time—several more weeks—is usually taken in processing the claim, and issuing checks in payment.

While most claims are processed routinely within a few weeks of their receipt, some are questioned, or are returned for further information. Therefore, a portion of claims will be set aside and delayed. Similarly, providers have different billing cycles. Some may bill immediately, or within a few days of performing a service. Others might produce invoices weekly, or on some other schedule. Whatever the schedule, there will be exceptions: some invoices will be delayed, for one reason or another.

As with any set of activities involving large numbers of events or cases, a pattern can be observed.

Recognizing the time patterns in claims records, actuaries have set up various methods for estimating the ultimate amount of claims, that is, the "completed" claims for any given period of exposure.

For Annual Statements to Insurance Departments, financial results for a year ended December 31 must usually be filed by March 1 or April 1, and a process of estimation is a necessary part of stating the costs for the year.

Unpaid claims are usually referred to as "IBNR", which means *Incurred But Not Reported* claims. To be precise, though, a distinction should be drawn between "IBNR"—unreported claims—and "IBNP", which refers to *Incurred But Not Paid* claims. IBNR is used when the value of all claims received is known, and an estimate is needed only for those which have *not been received*.

So "IBNR" only relates to claims which have not been received. It is based in data showing the pattern of time between the date of service and the receipt of the paperwork by the health plan. If "IBNR" is listed as part of the claims liability of a health plan, there must be a separate account of the balance of unpaid claims—those received but in the course of processing. (The latter are commonly referred to as RBUC, pronounced "rebuck", which likely refers to *Received But Un Completed*.)

To incorporate all claims liability in a single estimate, it is common to use IBNP for reporting purposes. This, of course, is based on data on the time lag between the date of service and the date of payment. In mature systems, this generally forms a regular pattern, allowing an accurate estimate of the total.

Whether for "IBNP" or "IBNR", the method of estimation is essentially the same: a pattern of claims payment (or receipt) is compiled, reflecting past experience, and the assumption is made that the current flow of claims will follow the past pattern. Thus, for example, it might be observed that, by the end of the month in which a service occurred, 10% will have been paid, by the end of the first month following, 60%, by the end of the second month following, 80%, etc. The percentages cited are referred to as "completion factors", i.e. the percent of the ultimate total complete at a given point in time. If, for example, $1,000,000 has been paid and the completion factor is 60%, this points to ultimate claims of $1,666,667 ($1,000,000 divided by .60) and to an unpaid liability of $666,667 ($1,666,667 minus $1,000,000). The underlying data is generally referred to as a "lag study", or "lag analysis", in that the object is to observe the pattern of time lags in receiving and/or paying claims.

While straightforward mathematical methods are used in estimating claims liabilities, it should be noted that, in regular application, the process of estimating claims liabilities takes skill and experience. Errors and misjudgments are frequently made. The path of health plan history is littered with the remains of those which have underestimated their ultimate claims liabilities. Many former health plan executives can date the ends of their leadership careers to a misjudgment (or an overoptimistic estimate) of total claims expenses. It cannot be said too strongly: the ability to do the arithmetic, to run a computer program, or to apply a formula does not equate to the ability to discern the right answer. That is what actuaries do. Their independence, and the requirements of their profession, support an objective view. That is why estimates of claims liabilities, in Annual Statements to regulators, must be certified by a qualified actuary.

PART VII

EXPERIENCE RATING

A. OVERVIEW—CHOICE OF METHODS

B. DATA REQUIREMENTS

C. CREDIBILITY

D. ILLUSTRATIVE FORMULAS AND WORKSHEETS

E. PRESENTATION AND FEEDBACK

A. OVERVIEW—CHOICE OF METHODS

Experience rating means that renewal rates, for each group, are based on a record of that group's experience. Thus a "high-cost group" (or low) identifies itself as such through the record of costs of care for its members. The experience-rating method used by a health plan incorporates a structured approach for determining how much of the group's past experience is to be considered predictive, or credible, for purposes of setting future rates. A record of past experience is interpreted to create a serviceable measure for setting future rates.

In all cases, a deliberate, structured, step-by-step process is involved.

Experience rating methods, or mechanisms, or formulas, are part of a health plan's rate filing with insurance departments. The methods filed are expected to be used uniformly, on all groups to which they apply. The methods, or formulas, determine what the rates will be—and thus are fully as important as any numeric value which may be included in a rate filing.

The main regulatory requirement is simple and universal: that the method filed, when applied to the data, will produce the renewal rates which are quoted. In other words, no special deals, no deviations from the formula.

A distinction can be drawn between two general approaches to the matter of adjusting rates for experience. One, which may be called the "traditional" experience-rating approach, is expressed in terms of the PMPM costs for the group, credibility factors, trends, and, from these, predicted costs or revenue requirements for the specific group.

Another follows the "Adjusted Community Rating" or "ACR" approach cited in the Federal HMO Act, and in many State laws. Here the key element is a prediction, based on experience, of the *relative cost* of the specific group compared to the average cost for all groups covered by the health plan. The result is expressed as a multiple of the standard rate, or community rate.

These two general approaches will usually produce similar results for a given subscriber group. The differences generally concern the data requirements, the ways in which the calculations are carried out, and the ways in which results are communicated to subscriber groups. We will discuss each of these approaches, and illustrate their application.

B. DATA REQUIREMENTS

"Traditional" experience rating depends upon an accurate record of claims expenses. That is, the basis of calculation—and the basis of explanations of results to subscriber groups—is a direct record of incurred expenses: the exact amounts.

An adjusted community rate (ACR) method, by contrast, can work on the basis of any valid measure of comparative costs. It is *not necessarily* based on complete experience data, or on direct measures of costs.

For example, the "traditional" approach would adjust the inpatient hospital part of the rate based on the precise costs incurred for hospitalization for each particular group, the ACR approach could work based simply on measures of bed days/1000 for the group and for the health plan as a whole, with the results expressed as a ratio: e.g. 1.10, 1.02, 0.95, etc.

Any experience rating approach must be carried out with full disclosure of the method and the supporting data. In turn, subscriber groups, particularly the larger ones, represented by skilled consultants, can be expected to challenge or test the validity of the data, in any way they can. In the process, they are likely to demand full documentation of costs: either claims-level data, or a summary which identifies utilization rates and unit costs.

It follows that if a health plan does not wish to reveal details of its provider reimbursement arrangements, or if it knows of system difficulties which stand in the way of presenting a full accounting of expenses for each group, it may find that a "traditional" experience rating approach would be hard to work with. Instead, an ACR approach, using ratios, might be more acceptable to the plan, if not to subscriber groups.

C. CREDIBILITY

The key concept in experience rating is credibility, or the degree to which the group-specific experience data is considered to be predictive. It is a function of the number of exposures: the size of the group and the frequency of the events.

Credibility is generally expressed in percentage terms: if a group's experience is considered to be 100% credible, it is fully predictive, if 50%, half-way, etc. If the group-specific percentage is less than 100%, the other part of the equation has to do with experience of the plan as a whole, or another representation of "standard" experience. For example, if a group's hospital experience is 250 days/1000/year, and the plan average is 300/1000, a 50% credibility factor would call for a 50/50 blend, producing a "credibility-adjusted" measure of 275 days per 1000. If the group is large enough so that its experience is considered to be 90% credible, for example, then the credibility-adjusted rate is (.90 x 250) + (.10 x 300) or 255 days/1000.

Credibility can be said to express the degree to which chance is *not* considered to be an explanation for the group-specific experience. It was observed in Part II that the range of likely variation in any element of experience is related to "exposure" which is the product of time and:

- The frequency of the event or service; and,
- The size of the group.

It follows that various elements of experience have different degrees of credibility. Frequent events or services, like physician office visits and the filling of drug prescriptions, are highly credible. That is, experience over a relatively short period of time can be considered to be a reliable prediction of future experience for such services. The rate of office visits, usually occurring at the rate of about 3500-4000 per 1000 persons per year, has a normal variance of only about 5% (plus or minus) for a group of 1,000 members, 7% for 500 members, 15% for 100. But hospitalization experience is *not* fully credible for most groups. Because hospital admissions are infrequent, chance is a significant element in determining utilization for all but the largest groups: the normal "swing" is about 35% (plus or minus) for a 1000-member group; it gets to be negligible, about 4%, for a group of 100,000 members.

In group insurance practice generally, specific mathematical determinations concerning credibility usually give way to judgments about what will be considered to be 100% credible. For example, it may be decided that overall experience for 1000 persons for a year, or perhaps 1000 contracts, will be considered—or deemed to be—fully credible, with the credibility percentages scaled according to membership: if 100% at 1000, then 50% at 500, etc.

Such measures of a credibility used in experience rating are arbitrary, and are meant to reflect a reasonable or serviceable measure, recognizing that the object is not mathematical precision but rather an acceptable tool.

Credibility factors are illustrated as follows for three broad kinds of health care services.

	Factor	"Full Credibility"
Hospital Care	$\sqrt{.00066667 \times n}$	1500 Member Years
Ambulatory Services	$\sqrt{.00133334 \times n}$	750 Member Years
Prescription Drugs	$\sqrt{.00400 \times n}$	250 Member Years

That is, the measure of credibility is the square root of the factors shown times the number of members. The factors are chosen as those which would result in 100% credibility (or a factor of 1.00) at a given level of enrollment. These factors reflect *judgments* as to the number of members for which experience—for this purpose—is *considered to be* 100% credible: 1500 members for hospital care services, 750 members for ambulatory services, and 250 members for prescription drugs. Such a set of factors is illustrated below.

Membership	Hospital (.00066667)	Ambulatory Services (.00133334)	Rx (.00400)
50	18.26%	25.82%	44.72%
100	25.82	36.51	63.25
150	31.62	44.72	77.46
200	36.51	51.64	89.44
250	40.82	57.74	100.00
500	57.74	81.65	100.00
750	70.71	100.00	100.00
1000	81.65	100.00	100.00
1250	91.29	100.00	100.00
1500 +	100.00	100.00	100.00

As an example, the following shows credibility factors reflecting another set of judgments: that the standards for presumed "full credibility" would be set twice as high.

Membership	Hospital (.00033334)	Ambulatory Services (.00066667)	Rx (.00200)
50	12.91%	18.26%	31.62%
100	18.26	25.82	44.72
150	22.36	31.62	54.77
200	25.82	36.51	63.25
250	28.87	40.82	70.71
500	40.83	57.74	100.00
750	50.00	70.71	100.00
1000	57.74	81.65	100.00
1250	64.55	91.29	100.00
1500	70.71	100.00	100.00
2000	81.65	100.00	100.00
2500	91.29	100.00	100.00
3000	100.00	100.00	100.00

A consideration in choice of such "working" credibility factors is the practice of other carriers active in the area. This may be learned from brokers and consultants, and, possibly, from rate filings (if the filing with the formula or method can be located). A search through recent rate filings for credibility factors and experience rating formulas may not be productive, since often these will be found to have been filed in the distant past, and maintained unchanged over long periods of time. Also, some formulas can be complex, and may not be described with clarity.

D. ILLUSTRATIVE FORMULAS AND WORKSHEETS

Some practical points about procedure can be made through review of two worksheets, one concerning traditional experience rating, the other, adjusted community rating, or ACR.

The worksheet provided in this section concerns experience rating: a prediction based on the experience of a particular group, as modified by credibility factors.

This worksheet is constructed to take into account overall or total experience for a group. It serves for illustration. A strong argument can be made that, because of differing completion factors and credibility factors, an experience-rating analysis should incorporate at least three segments: hospital care, ambulatory services, and prescription drugs. This can be readily done in a computer spreadsheet. The format illustrated here incorporates all necessary steps, in sequence, and it all fits on one page.

The first set of entries, identifying the periods of time involved and the number of member months in the experience period, etc. are essential in that they identify the specific, precise measures to be used in the process.

Trending is from the experience period (or observation period) to the rating period, and generally is carried out in terms of the number of months, from the mid-point or the experience period to the mid-point of the rate period.

The date that the experience data was compiled indicates which completion factor (or factors) should be used, by reference to the health plans' regular claims liability estimates. For example, it might be observed that overall experience for a year, run precisely at the end of that year, would be considered 82% complete. If run to include claims paid one month following the end of the year, it would be 90% complete, two months, 95%, three months, 97%.

As observed elsewhere in this volume, such factors are specific to each plan, to each line of business, and can be developed for each type of service. These factors also change, with changes in the speed of claims submission, processing, and payment. So reference to relevant and contemporary factors is essential: the sources should be documented; use of "rules of thumb" is inadvisable. In all events, the factors used for experience rating purposes should be the same as used by the health plan for its financial reports.

An appropriate credibility factor needs to be entered, reflecting the size of the group, expressed in terms of the average membership during the experience period. This requires reference to the filed factors. Again, this is not a matter for discretion or judgment to be exercised during the process of determining rates for any account. There is a wide range of possibilities in what factors may be filed, and the filed factors can be changed. But in any application, the filed factors must be used.

The "benefit factor" in this worksheet is used if the program of benefits is to change, from the experience period to the rating period. This is based on the relative costliness of the entire program of benefits as measured by the standard rates, or "book rates" in the rate filing. For example, if office visit copays are to be increased $5 (for example from $5 per visit to $10 for primary care, and from $10 to $15 for specialty visits) and the value of that reduces the book capitation rate from $160 to $158 PMPM; the difference in standard rates may be measured as a 1.25% decline, from a factor of 1.0000 to a factor of 0.9875.

EXPERIENCE RATING WORKSHEET

Group Name: _____
Rating Period: _____ through _____ (Midpoint) _____
Experience Period: _____ through _____ (Midpoint) _____
Experience Data Compiled on _____ Completion Factor _____
Exp. Period Average Membership _____ Credibility Factor _____
Benefit Factor—Exp. Period _____ (A) Benefit Factor—Rating Period _____ (B)
Pooling Attachment Point $_____ (PMPY) Pooling Factor _____

#

1.	Paid Claims—Experience Period	$_____	Claims Record
2.	Less Claims Amounts over Attachment Point	$_____	Claims Record
3.	Net Paid Claims	$_____	1 - 2 = 3
4.	Completion Factor	$_____	Input Data Above
5.	Net Incurred Claims	$_____	3 / 4 = 5
6	Member Months—Experience Period	$_____	Membership Record
7.	Net Incurred Claims (PMPM)	$_____	5 / 6 = 7
8.	Pooling Factor	$_____	Input Data Above
9.	Gross Incurred Claims (PMPM)	$_____	7 / 8 = 9
10.	Credibility Factor	$_____	Input Data Above
11.	Book Rate (PMPM)	$ _____	Look Up
12.	Credibility-Adjusted Incurred Claims (PMPM)	$_____	(10 x 9) + (1.0 - 10 x 11) = 12
13.	Capitation Expense-Experience Period (PMPM)	$_____	
14.	Total Health Services Expense—Experience Period (PMPM)	$_____	12 + 13 = 14
15.	Trend Factor	$_____	
16.	Trended Health Services Expense (PMPM)	$_____	14 x 15 = 16
17.	Benefit Change Factor	$_____	
18.	Modified Projected Health Services Expenses	$_____	16 x 17 = 18
19.	Loading	$_____	% of Total Revenue Requirement
20.	Commissions	$_____	% of Total Revenue Requirement
21.	Revenue Requirement (PMPM)	$_____	18 / [1.0 - (19 + 20)] = 21
22.	Revenue at Current Rates (PMPM)	$_____	Look up
23.	Adjustment Factor	$_____	21 / 22 = 23

#

The following observations are numbered in accordance with the entries on the worksheet.

1. *Paid Claims/Experience Period.* This is a gross amount. Care should be taken to assure that the amount entered is consistent with other accounts of paid claims provided to groups.
2. *Less Claims Amount Over Pooling Attachment Point.* The object here is to remove "catastrophic claims" from the equation. These occur randomly, with a large element of luck, and thus the costs of these "jumbo" claims may not reflect the underlying cost characteristics of the group. This level can be varied: for small groups it might be, say, $25,000; for the very largest groups, perhaps $100,000 or even $250,000.

   A common error at this point is to remove the entire amount for those persons who exceed the attachment point. Only the amounts over the attachment point should be removed.
3. *Net Paid Claims.* This is simply the result of subtracting the amounts over the attachment point, for the "jumbo" or high-cost claims, from the total.
4. *Completion Factors.* This is simply the factor entered above, reflecting the time covered in the experience period, and the time on which the experience data was compiled. This is generally expressed as a number, or percentage, reflecting the extent to which claims are complete. This should be the same factor used for financial reporting purposes by the health plan.
5. *Net Incurred Claims.* Net paid claims divided by the completion factor yields net incurred claims. For example, $1,000,000 divided by .91 equals $1,098,901.10.
6. *Member Months—Experience Period.* This is the denominator related to the numerator entered as "net incurred claims", in other words, the number of member months for the same group, and for the same period of time. Adjustments for retroactivity, etc., if any, should be reflected in the denominator, so that there is no question about the accuracy and appropriateness of the PMPM result, expressed in the next line.
7. *Net Incurred Claims PMPM.* This is the amount of incurred claims expressed on a PMPM basis.
8. *Pooling Factor.* A continuance table, for the class of business as a whole, should indicate the value of claims, above and below an "attachment

point". The claims up to the attachment point include two parts: all the claims for members with costs up to the attachment point, and costs up to the attachment point for all others. The "pooling" factor as used here represents the portion of total claims *under* the attachment point: for example, the value of claims up to $100,000 per person per year representing, say, 92% of total costs, over $100,000, the remaining 8%.

9. *Gross Incurred Claims (PMPM)*. This is the product, after application of the pooling factor. In other words, it is a measure of the total claims, including the portion that is pooled. For example, if the pooling factor is .92, and net incurred claims (Line 7) are $200 PMPM, then gross incurred claims will be $200 / .92 or $217.39.

10. *Credibility Factor*. This reflects the filed credibility factor, appropriate for the average membership of the group in the experience period. It can be described as the weight to be given to the group's own experience, with the balance given to the book rate.

11. *Book Rate PMPM*. This is obtained by referring to the filed rates, i.e. the standard rates for the precise benefit program which the group has had during the experience period.

12. *Credibility-Adjusted Incurred Claims (PMPM)*. This represents a blend, using the credibility factor, of the net incurred claims (Line 7) and the book rate (Line 11). The incurred claims PMPM, in Line 7, are multiplied by the applicable credibility factor, (.60, for sake of an example) and the book rate (Line 11) is multiplied by the reciprocal of the credibility factor (1.0 - .60, or .40). The products of these two multiplications are summed and the result is entered in Line 12. As an example, assume that the net incurred claims PMPM is $220, given 60% weight, while the book rate is $200, given 40% weight. Then, 60% of the group's net incurred claims plus 40% of the book rate are added together to indicate a credibility-adjusted incurred claims amount, in Line 12, of, for example, $212 PMPM.

13. *Capitation Expense / Experience Period (PMPM)*. If a portion of the services have been capitated, during the expense period, and not included in the claims record, the PMPM value of such services should be added at this point.

14. *Total Health Services Expense / Experience Period (PMPM)*. This is the sum of Lines 12 and 13, non-capitated and capitated expenses.

15. *Trend Factor*. This is the factor which expresses the expected annual rate of increase. It is *not* a reflection of ad hoc judgment, specific to the particular group. Rather, it is a reflection of the overall trend cited by the health plan in its filed rates. If, as is usual, there are different trend

factors for prescription drugs and for other benefits, a blended rate can be structured for use at this point. For example, if 20% of the book value of the benefit package were represented by drug benefits, at an annual rate of increase of (for example) 14%, and if 80% represented other benefits at an annual rate of 8%, the blended trend rate would be 9.2%. (Alternatively, as suggested earlier, a separate worksheet specifically for drug benefits could be used. This would—in most cases—not include the steps in this worksheet involving completion factors and credibility factors, since drug claims are usually complete within a month, and credibility factors are usually considered to be 100%.)

16. *Trended Health Services Expense (PMPM).* This is the product of the trend factor (Line 15) applied to total health services expense (Line 14).
17. *Benefit Change Factor.* This is obtained from the rate filing or book rates. It reflects the relative cost, as expressed in the book rates, for one benefit program or another. If the benefit program is to become less costly, or less generous, the factor would be less than one; if the changes are in the direction of increasing benefits, or reducing copays, the factor would be a positive one, e.g. more than 1.00.
18. *Modified Projected Health Services Expenses.* This reflects the effect of the benefit change factor.
19 & 20. *Loading and Commissions.* In this worksheet, these are each expressed as a percentage of the total revenue requirement for health services. Some plans express loadings, or portions of them, as per-capita amounts.
21. *Revenue Requirement (PMPM).* This reflects the projected health services expense, (Line 18) grossed up to include loading and commissions (Lines 19 & 20).
22. *Revenue at Current Rates (PMPM).* This is obtained by dividing the total premium revenue, for a recent period, by the number of member months for the same period. It reflects the *actual* per-capita yield from the premiums in effect, for the group in question. (This may be substantially different from the per-capita yield which had been intended or projected for the group, and will not ordinarily be the same exact amount.)
23. *Adjustment Factor.* This "bottom line" represents the percentage by which the existing rates are to be changed. Generally speaking, existing rate ratios are maintained: the percentage adjustment applies to each rate tier. (This bypasses the step of constructing the premium rates from the capitation rates, based on contract mix, contract size, and rate ratios, as described in Part VIII: Premium Rate Development.)

—#—

An ACR worksheet is illustrated on the next page. It is constructed to take into account four years of experience and to present the results in terms of weighted average, credibility-adjusted cost ratios for three elements of experience: ambulatory services, inpatient hospital services, and prescription drugs.

The resulting factors express the extent to which experience indicates that the subject group is more or less costly than the average for all groups in the rate class. These factors are applied to the components of the community rate, as adjusted for copays and other benefit variations, to produce the health services revenue requirement for the group.

Credibility factors to be used are shown in the lower left-hand portion of the illustrative worksheet.

ILLUSTRATIVE ACR WORKSHEET

Group Name _____ Renewal Date _____

Experience Years End on: (1) _____ (2) _____ (3) _____ (4) _____

DEVELOPMENT OF EXPERIENCE RATIOS

		Ambulatory			IP Hospital			Rx	
	Average Membership	Exp. Ratio	Factor (A)	Cred. Adj. Ratio*	Exp. Ratio	Factor (B)	Cred. Adj. Ratio*	Exp. Ratio	Factor (C)	Cred. Adj. Ratio*
Year 1	___	___	___	___	___	___	___	___	___	___
Year 2	___	___	___	___	___	___	___	___	___	___
Year 3	___	___	___	___	___	___	___	___	___	___
Year 4	___	___	___	___	___	___	___	___	___	___
Total / Wt. Avg.	___			___			___			___

* Credibility adjusted ratio: Products of credibility factors appropriate to average membership and type of service time's experience ratio plus reciprocal of such factor times 1.00.
Example: 70% x 1.10 + 30% x 1.00 = 1.07.

CREDIBILITY FACTORS

Average Membership	(A) Ambulatory	(B) IP Hospital	(C) Rx
50 – 99	30%	20%	50%
100 – 249	50	30	75
250 – 499	70	50	100
500 – 749	90	70	100
750 – 1000	100	100	100
1000 +	100	100	100

APPLICATION

	Cred. Adj. Experience Ratios	Community Rate Component PMPM	Product Adjusted Community Rate (PMPM)
Ambulatory	___	$ ___	$ ___
I.P. Hospital	___	___	___
Rx	___	___	___
		$ ___	$ ___

The process of completing the worksheet involves looking up and applying experience ratios which would be tabulated for all groups in the rate class. Reference also needs to be made to exposure: the average membership (or, alternatively, total member months) in each policy year. The experience ratios are applied to the credibility factors to produce credibility-adjusted ratios for each service type, for each year. From these, a weighted average is produced, reflecting experience over the most recent four years, for that group. The following illustrates this.

Year	Average Membership	Cred. Adjusted Cost Ratio
Latest	1000	1.052
+1	800	1.030
+2	850	.925
+3	900	.951
Total/Wtd. Average	3550	0.991

That is, the weighted average of the ratios, in this case, is 0.991.

Many practitioners believe that more recent experience is more relevant, and has greater predictive power. A "time-weight" can be added to the membership-weight. In the following example, the latest year has 50% weight, and each earlier year has lower weight.

Year	Avg. Membership	Time Weight	Product	Cred. Adjusted Ratio
Latest	1000	.50	500	1.052
+1	800	.30	240	1.030
+2	850	.10	85	.925
+3	900	.10	90	.951
	3550	1.00	915	1.024

As can be seen from this brief example, an ACR process can be carried out with simple measures of relative experience. The product of the ACR calculations is simply a factor, plus or minus, which is multiplied by the standard or "book" rate for the benefit plan offered to produce an appropriate level of charge for a group.

E. PRESENTATION AND FEEDBACK

The worksheets and supporting documentation referred to in the preceding section should, ideally, be clear enough so that they can be presented to subscriber groups, and their representatives, as support for upcoming rate adjustments.

Essentially the process of presentation is part of the rate development process. This involves decisions on formats. It also involves strict attention to the accuracy and consistency of the data used in the rating calculation.

Staff training is also a consideration. The finance and/or underwriting staffs of a health plan need not be involved in the presentation of each rate renewal, and in discussions with subscriber groups. That is usually part of the job of the marketing department or the account services staff. The people involved with servicing group accounts should be trained to understand the rate calculations, to present them in a way that is understandable, and to answer most questions.

While it can be expected that most requests for substantial rate adjustments will meet with some resistance, an objective and understandable presentation is more likely to be accepted. If representatives of subscriber groups perceive the use of a "black box" approach: something they cannot understand or which is not clearly justified, this is likely to impel them to attempt to negotiate, and/or to shop for a better rate. If the perception is allowed that the rates really derive from someone's opinion (and/or that the description of the rate calculation is mumbo-jumbo), subscriber groups will be compelled to object.

There are some markets, and some market segments, in which negotiation of rates is traditional, and expected. While much can be said on this subject, the essential point is that insurance laws, which require non-discrimination in rate setting, effectively limit the scope in which discretion can be exercised.

The essential requirement, as described in Part I of this volume, is that if any exception or concession is granted to any subscriber group, the carrier must extend the same advantage to any similarly-situated group.

As a practical matter, this requirement can be readily met in the case of very large groups, i.e. those which can be characterized as unique. So, for example, a lower retention for a unique 25,000-member group could be justified by measurably lower costs for sales and for premium accounting. So a precedent, applicable to groups of that size, would be workable. The adjustment, or concession, would apply to all such groups. But if a 100-member group, one of many similar groups, demands a lower overhead charge, the health plan could not find a legitimate basis to accede, without reducing its charges for all such groups.

Feedback in rate discussions might be characterized as part of negotiations. But it can also be said to involve the process of bringing additional factors to the attention of health plan representatives: "You ought to take account of . . .". This is a legitimate activity, especially in situations where the rating formulas are relatively complex.

For the experience-rating or ACR methods illustrated in this chapter, feedback and discussion would primarily be concerned with the accuracy of the data used. A subscriber group representative would be acting responsibly (and not simply creating a nuisance) in seeking to verify that the input data is appropriate and thereby to test the results.

Assuming that the input data is correct, a robust system for rate adjustment is one which, in effect, anticipates the questions which will be asked. Presentation should generally contain these elements, in order: (1) method used; (2) data; (3) application of data to method; (4) results. This logically builds to a conclusion that the facts produce the result—and that a different result would have to come from a different method, or different data.

A final note on the subject of rate presentations is that subscriber group representatives, involved in the process of rate renewals, need to acquire the facts so that, in turn, they can explain and interpret the rate action to the responsible parties. A representative has to be mindful of how he or she will "report back" on the rate discussions. While some subscriber group representatives may prefer to report a negotiating success—that the health plan had "backed down" and accepted a lower premium—the next best thing is a cogent and convincing explanation of how the rate is justified.

PART VIII

PREMIUM RATE DEVELOPMENT

A. PREMIUM RATES: MARKET DETERMINANTS AND OPTIONS

B. PREMIUM RATE MECHANICS

C. DATA FOR PREMIUM RATE DEVELOPMENT

D. PROBLEMS WITH PREMIUMS

E. RATES FOR SMALL GROUPS

A. PREMIUM RATES: MARKET DETERMINANTS AND OPTIONS

Group health insurance in the U.S. was first developed around a two-tier rate structure: individual rates and family rates.

Early methods of premium collection and accounting demanded simplicity, and a two-tier rate structure met that need.

With the increase in the number of families with two wage-earners, it became common for family members to be covered twice: a wife and children could be covered under the husband's coverage; while the husband and children would be covered, again, through the wife's group.

So long as the employers were paying most of the cost of coverage, and so long as rates were based on experience, such multiple coverage didn't matter much, and was largely ignored by employers. Rules on Coordination of Benefits, adopted by the insurance industry in the 1960s, established which plan would pay for each episode of care.

But, with higher costs, and the increase in employee contributions to the cost of group health coverage, a demand arose for additional tiers or groupings. This was underlined, for HMOs, by the fact that, unlike traditional carriers, they did not operate on a cost-plus basis, returning surplus funds.

The components of the commonly-used tiers are usually as follows.

Five Tier	Four Tier	Three Tier	Two Tier
Single	Single	Single	Single
Husband/Wife	Husband/Wife	Two Person	Family
Parent/ Child	Parent/Child(ren)		
Parent/Children		Family	
Family	Family		

In general, the greater the level of employee participation in cost, the more demand there will be for multiple tiers. This furthers equity and acceptance: a parent with one child will have, in a five-tier structure, a rate lower than that for a multiple-child family. Those with "split" families (in terms of coverage) will not be paying rates which include the costs for the family member who is covered through other employment.

The usual rule in choosing which tier structure to use is: "Follow the market"! There are geographic patterns in rate structures. In the industrial Northeast, two-tier and three-tier rate structures have been in place for many years, are accepted, and are routinely used even in small-group situations where four-tier or five-tier rates would make sense.

It is possible to have a "one-tier" rate structure, or a "super-composite", i.e. a per-employee rate, and some employers have required that, for the sake of administrative simplicity.

A sixth "tier" is sometimes added, covering dependent children who may be enrolled separately from their parents. Another variation—producing a seventh tier—could include a rate for dependent parents, who are sometimes included as dependents in work-based coverage.

It would be possible—theoretically—for premiums to be charged on a per-capita basis. But this has not happened in the private market. (Per capita rates are the norm, however, in government programs—Medicare and Medicaid.)

In all events, the object of the premium-setting process is to translate the health plan's per-capita revenue requirements into the suitable market format.

B. PREMIUM RATE MECHANICS

The premium-setting process aims to assure that the premiums yield enough to match the revenue requirements represented by the per capita budget.

The usual procedure in premium rate development is illustrated in the following four steps.

(1) *The monthly capitation rate or "Revenue Requirement" is determined.* This involves the time period of the contract, the particular plan of benefits, the demographics of the group, and/or the group's unique revenue requirements as indicated by experience data. The rate filing sets forth the basis for the revenue requirement and the rules for application to a particular group.

(2) *Decisions are made as to the number of tiers and the rate ratios.* In the example below, we illustrate the use of:

- A 3-tier rate;
- A 1:2:3 ratio—the family rate is 3 times the single rate, and the couple rate is twice the single rate. The "rate ratio" is sometimes referred to as the "slope", or the "slope of the rates".

(3) *The contract-mix and family size characteristics of the group are noted.* In the example below:

- 40% of the covered employees in a group are expected to have

single contracts, 10% two-person contracts, and the remaining 50% to have family contracts.
- The average family size is 4.0 persons.

(4) *The arithmetic is done to produce the rates.* This involves three steps:

   (a) Development of a factor which defines the difference between the capitation rate and the single rate. (This is referred to as a "step-up factor" because, usually, the single rate is higher than the capitation rate.)
   (b) Application of the factor to produce the single rate.
   (c) Application of the rate ratios to produce the other rates.

The development of the "step-up factor" is illustrated as follows.

Type	Mix	Ratio	Size	Mix x Ratio	Mix x Size
Single	40%	1.0	1.0	0.40	0.40
Couple	10%	2.0	2.0	0.20	0.20
Family	50%	3.0	4.0	1.50	2.00
	100%			2.10	2.60

2.60 divided by 2.10 = 1.2380952

That is, a factor (in this case 1.2380952) is calculated, which, when multiplied by the capitation rate, produces the single rate. The chosen multiples of the single rate create the two-person and family rates. (In this example, the couple rate is twice the single rate and the family rate is three times the single rate.)

The rate development process can be further illustrated by assuming a $230 capitation rate. First the step-up factor is applied to get the single rate; then the single rate is multiplied by the rate ratios to produce the 2-person and family rates.

1.2380952	x	$230	=	$284.76	Single rate
$284.76	x	x 2.0	=	$569.52	2-Person rate
$284.76	x	x 3.0	=	$854.29	Family rate

If the rates are calculated "by hand" (not in a regularly-used computer program) it is a good idea to test them to make sure that they actually yield the intended per capita amount. This goes like this:

RATING AND UNDERWRITING FOR HEALTH PLANS

Type	Proportion	Rate
Single	40%	$284.76
2-Person	10%	569.52
Family	50%	854.29
	100%	$598.00

The weighted average revenue per contract is $598.00. When that is divided by average contract size (2.60), the product is $230.00. This proves that the rate calculation "worked".

—#—

The process described may seem convoluted. But it can be explained in terms of the fact that the revenue requirement for the group (number of persons times the capitation rate) needs to be accommodated *within the constraints of the rate ratios*.

Visualized in terms of (for example) 100 employees and contracts, we see that if the average contract size is 2.6, 100 contracts will contain 260 people, and the rates need to produce enough money for each of these. If the per-capita revenue requirement is $230, then $59,800 per month (260 x $230) needs to be generated each month from the rates.

	Number of Contracts	Contract Size	Number of Persons
Single	40	1.0	40
Couple	10	2.0	20
Family	50	4.0	200
	100	2.6	260

At the same time, if the ratio of rates is to be 1:2:3, then only 210 *rate units* are available:

Contract Type	Number of Contracts	Rate Ratio	Number of "Rate Units"
Single	40	1.0	40
Couple	10	2.0	20
Family	50	3.0	150
	100	2.1	210

If 210 "rate units" are to generate revenue for 260 persons—or if $59,800 per month is to be raised from 210 "rate units"—then it can be seen that each "unit" must be worth $59,800 divided by 210, or $284.76. That amount becomes the single rate: the same as was shown on the previous page as a product of the "formula".

—#—

While the "step-up factor" above is taken to 7 decimal places, and computers add more in processing the numbers, it is perhaps worthwhile to observe that practical application can involve some rounding and simplification. Adequate rates are the goal, not necessarily mathematical elegance.

—#—

To recap, the rate setting process can be viewed as being entered on a worksheet, like this one:

	(A) Mix x Size	(B) Mix x Ratio
Single	____% x 1.0	____% x 1.0
2-Person	____% x 2.0	____% x ____ (Ratio)
Family	____% x ____(Size)	____% x ____ (Ratio)
Sums—Wt. Avg.	100.0% ____ (A)	100.0% ____ (B)

(A) ____ Divided by (B) ____ = (C) ____
                                        Multiplier (or step-up factor)

____ x $ ____ = $ ____ Single Rate
Multiplier (or step-up factor) Capitation Rate

Single Rate x ____ = $ ____ 2-Person Rate
              Ratio

Single Rate x ____ = $ ____ Family Rate
              Ratio

RATING AND UNDERWRITING FOR HEALTH PLANS

With the numbers filled in, the worksheet would look like this:

	Mix x Size	Mix x Ratio
Single	50% x 1.0	50% x 1.0
2-Person	10% x 2.0	10% x 2.1
Family	40% x 4.0	40% x 3.2
Sums—Wt. Avg.	100.0% 2.30 (A)	100.0% 1.99 (B)

(A) 2.30 Divided by (B) 1.99 = (C) 1.15577889 (1.1558)
Multiplier (or step-up factor)

Multiplier (or step-up factor) 1.1558 x $240 = $277.39 Single Rate
Capitation Rate

Single Rate x 2.1 = $582.52 2-Person Rate
Ratio

Single Rate x 3.2 = $887.65 Family Rate
Ratio

An archaic approach, now rarely used, was to develop the premium rates using demographic factors, and then redistribute such rates to achieve the desired ratios. For example, the rates may be initially developed from the following cost weights and distribution of members by contract type:

Single Contract:	0.60 female	@ 1.250 x $200 =	$150.00
	0.40 male	@ 0.975 x $200 =	78.00
	1.00		$228.00
Family Contract:	1.00 female	@ 1.35 x $200 =	$270.00
	1.00 male	@ 0.975 x $200 =	195.00
	1.90 children	@ 0.65 x $200 =	247.00
	3.90		$712.00

RATING AND UNDERWRITING FOR HEALTH PLANS

The foregoing results in a ratio of 1:3.1228 ($712/$228), whereas a ratio of 1:2.90 is desired to match the rate ratios of competitive carriers. A reallocation to that market-appropriate ratio can be done as follows:

Contract Type	Distribution	Original Rate	Ratio	Desired Ratio
Single	40%	$228.00	1.0000	1.000
Family	60%	712.00	3.1228	2.900
Weighted Avg.	100%	$518.40	2.27368	2.140

2.27368 divided by 2.140 = 1.062467 (factor)

REALLOCATION

Contract Type	Distribution	Original	Factor	Product	Ratio
Single	40%	$228.00	1.062467	$242.24	1.0
Family	60%	—	—	$702.50 *	2.9
	100%				

* 2.9 x $242.24 = $702.50

This works. But it might be said to represent the long way around to the goal of a market-appropriate rate.

C. DATA FOR PREMIUM RATE DEVELOPMENT

While the arithmetic in premium rate development can be done in a few minutes—or in milliseconds by a computer—gathering the necessary information for a new rate quote is another matter.

Relevant data includes, for each group:

- Data, or a judgment, about the likely *contract distribution*—mainly the percentage of single enrollees;
- Facts, or a judgment, on *family contract size*;
- *Rate ratios* in competing or dual choice products.

Contract mix and family size data involves an element of judgment. First, the relevant facts (concerning the employees) are always changing—slowly and subtly for large groups, perhaps very quickly for small groups. Second, in situations where employees have a choice, it is necessary to anticipate whether the characteristics of the people who actually enroll will mirror those of the group as a whole, or reflect some type of selection.

To adequately deal with this, an underwriter or rate-setter should know something about the characteristics of:

(a) The health plan enrollees from this particular employer;
(b) Its enrollees from similar employers;
(c) The entire work force (not just enrollees) from the particular employer; and,
(d) The entire work force (not just enrollees) from similar employers.

Industry-wide or multi-health plan studies of contract mix and family size might identify the usual characteristics by type of employer—such as office employees of the state, transit system workers, nurses and other hospital workers, teachers, bank employees, auto workers, etc.

Special note should be made of historical data for a particular account or subscriber group. A trend toward a greater family size or a higher family content is often noted as enrollment grows from year to year. If so, this should be reflected in a future projection.

Since it will not always be possible to make a confident prediction of contract mix and family size characteristics for a particular group, especially a small one, it is useful to approach this through a systematic, documented weighted average approach, i.e. "backing in" to a rate using a combination of data from several sources: the group itself, similar employers, all groups in the health plan.

Weights for each can be assigned, based on the judgment of the analyst or underwriter. An example of a set of such weights is as follows:

ILLUSTRATIVE WEIGHTS BY DATA SOURCE

Potential Contract Years of Exposure	Plan Enrollees from This Employer	All Employees of This Employer	Average of Similar Employers	All Groups in Health Plan
New Groups				
Under 100	—	—	—	100%
Over 100	—	25%	25%	50%
Existing Group				
Under 1000	25%	25%	25%	25%
Over 1000	50%	25%	25%	—
Over 2500	75%	25%	—	—
Over 5000	100%	—	—	—

While the application of such an approach can't guarantee an accurate prediction, it is more reliable than a guess or a hunch. The essential idea is to make the process of estimation systematic, based on such facts as are available and consistent. If a pure guess is allowed, it can be too easy to justify a conclusion which supports a lower "step-up factor" and a lower rate.

In situations where enrollment is voluntary, it is sometimes possible to agree with the employer—before the enrollment takes place—that an adjustment can be made, based on characteristics of those who actually enroll. This is likely to be acceptable if the extent of a possible upward adjustment is limited. The rate quote is then in a range, with the final rate—within the range—to depend on the contract mix and family size of the actual enrollment.

D. PROBLEMS WITH PREMIUMS

In many cases, health plans have failed to adopt—or enforce—sound policies regarding rate-setting. This has led to significant problems, including these:

(1) Inadequate yields;
(2) Narrow market scope;
(3) Inappropriate uses of flexibility;
(4) Instability of rates.

The matter of *inadequate yields* is obvious. If erroneous judgments are made about contract mix and family size, actual yields can be substantially different from those intended.

A method of assessing the adequacy of rates by group or account is simply to divide the monthly premium yield by the number of people covered, as in the illustration below. This will identify problem accounts. Starting with such an analysis, the health plan can determine a procedure or strategy for improving yields.

Group	Monthly Yield	Total Members	Per Capita Yield
0001	$21,250	85	$250.00
0002	85,575	350	244.50
0003	28,060	122	230.00

The second problem with premium rates might be characterized as *narrow market scope.*

Some time ago, health plans—operating under early interpretations of community rating rules—typically made a single set of assumptions about contract mix and family size, and a single decision regarding rating ratios. This produced "one rate for all", just like the early Blue Cross plans. But such rates do not fit all situations in the health plan. They are too much for some groups, too little for others.

If a carrier charges a single set of market rates, then its market is effectively restricted to those groups which:

(a) can afford the coverage; and,
(b) have contract-mix/family-size characteristics that will produce an adequate per-capita yield to the health plan.

While such a simple approach to rates has enabled many of the early plans to get started (and even to prosper) a narrow market definition will not sustain substantial growth in all situations. Rating formats have to work in a wide variety of circumstances. In many cases, historically, excessive rigidity was replaced by inappropriate flexibility.

This resulted in:

(a) inadequate yields;
(b) attraction of non-representative (generally more expensive) populations;
(c) unstable rates to subscriber groups.

This had understandable origins, including the following:

(a) The arithmetic for determining premium rates is readily done;
(b) Data on family size and contract mix is not always available, or it can be misused, or misinterpreted;
(c) There has been little sustained official surveillance of this area by state insurance departments;
(d) Competition is intense, prompting a search for an "edge".

It is relatively easy to "imagine" a high concentration of single contracts and a low family size, leading to understated rates. So if rates are set on the basis of hunches, one can be seen as being as good as another, and the stage can be set for inadequate rates.

Some health plans have practiced "aggressive pricing" by varying rating ratios and tiers, in an attempt to gain a short-term advantage.

A plan in a dual—or multiple—choice situation can set its rating ratios at variance with those of its competitors: whether intentionally or through inattention. The inevitable result will be disproportionate enrollment in the rate categories (single, couple, family, etc.) which receive a relative "bargain". This is illustrated in the following examples which start with the same capitation rate.

	Ratios		Rates	
EXAMPLE 1	Plan	Competitor	Plan	Competitor
Single	1.0	1.0	$297.14	$312.00
Couple	2.0	2.0	594.28	624.00
Family	3.0	2.8	891.42	873.60

(The plan, charging relatively more to families, charges relatively less to couples and singles.)

	Plan	Competitor	Plan	Competitor
EXAMPLE 2				
Single	1.0	1.0	$328.42	$283.63
Family	2.5	3.0	$821.05	$850.91

(Here the plan will be a relative bargain for families, while the competitor's rates appeal especially to single enrollees.)

The effect of all of this can be also influenced by the relative worth of the competing benefit packages. In general, however:

(1) Membership in the plan will *tend* to be skewed in the direction of the "bargain" offered;
(2) This compounds the task of prediction;
(3) The most prevalent result has been:

  (a) lower-than-anticipated revenue, or
  (b) higher-than-anticipated cost.

The main point to be made here is that the search for better rates is constant, and many propositions regarding rate tiers and ratios can be persuasively presented. Alternate rates, using different scenarios, can be readily calculated. There is, in fact, lots of room for strategic thinking. But each idea needs to be tested in terms of its likely results on: (a) per capita yield, and (b) the composition of the membership.

Changes in membership composition are subtle in terms of immediate effect but important—potentially serious—over the long run: persistent use of rate ratios favorable to singles can drive up the average age of the health plan's enrollment. If that happens, experience leads to higher per capita rates, which may not be competitive. This is a problem which can be solved, but it can take some time—and membership losses—before such a plan is "back on the track" with competitive rates.

Rate instability is a problem for smaller groups. This comes simply from the fact that contract mix characteristics can change, from rate year to rate year. In a group of, say, 20 employees, it would not be unusual to see the percentage of single enrollees varying considerably. For example, those may be 40% of employees (8 persons) in the first year, 55% (11 persons) in the second year, then down to, say, 35% (7 persons) in the third year, etc.

The problem is much less pronounced in larger groups: the routine fluctuations in employment and enrollment, for groups of, say, 200 or more, are not likely to have a serious impact on the average contract size and on the "step-up factor". For groups of 25 or fewer employees, routine changes in employment can have extreme effects on rates—if these are calculated group by group.

For smaller groups, then, this adds a reason for so-called "rate book" pricing: the age-banded rates described next. If a step-up factor is used for smaller groups, all concerned should understand that the step-up factor can change significantly from year to year, and that this will result in rate actions which are different from the progression of the underlying capitation rate. For example, a health plan's underlying capitation rate, or budget, could increase at, say, 10% per year, while changes in the contract mix and contract size characteristics of the group might dictate premium adjustments of substantially different magnitudes: say as low as 5% or as high as 20%.

In setting premiums, the keys to successful operation are:

— careful attention to the data used in the rate-setting process;
— regular monitoring of all amounts to assure that per capita income comes close to expectations and requirements.

This is a crucial part of a health plan's activity. Mistakes are easy to make, and can have a significant impact on revenue.

At the same time, most revenue shortfalls—if discovered—can possibly be remedied if employers can be brought to understand that the *real* revenue requirement is expressed in the capitation rate, and that the premium rates reflect only the means to collect them. In cases in which there are questions about the assumptions used in building premium rates, it is a good idea to share questions, and the worksheets, with employers. In that way they can more readily understand if an adjustment needs to be made.

Because premium rate-setting involves care in gathering facts, and judgment in interpreting them, it is a good idea—generally—to concentrate responsibility for this function in one person, or, in a large organization, several. Documentation is essential, not only because of the need to assign responsibility, but also to assure that the organization, through its staff members, can learn how to carry out this function successfully—so that the premium rates yield the required per-capita revenue.

E. RATES FOR SMALL GROUPS

What has been said so far in this Part mostly concerns premium rates for larger groups. Special rules and calculations apply to most small-group business.

In such groups, it is likely that a substantial part of the premiums will be paid by the employee. This, in the first place, calls for rates which are most specific to the enrollee, matching the employees' characteristics—in terms of age and contract type—as closely as possible.

In this regard:

- *Contract types* reflect the number of persons covered under a contract. Four tier or five tier rate structures are usual for small groups.
- *Age bands* reflect the age of the enrolled employee.

An example of an age-banded set of rates is as follows:

CONTRACT TYPE	AGE	FACTOR	MONTHLY PREMIUMS
Single			
	Under 30	0.9062	$ 226.55
	30-39	1.1242	$ 281.05
	40-49	1.2937	$ 323.43
	50-59	1.7226	$ 430.05
	60+	2.3327	$ 583.18
Employee & Spouse			
	Under 30	1.7230	$ 430.75
	30-39	2.1121	$ 528.03
	40-49	2.4867	$ 621.68
	50-59	3.3354	$ 833.85
	60+	4.4853	$1121.33
Parent & Child			
	Under 30	1.6133	$ 403.33
	30-39	1.8118	$ 452.95
	40-49	1.8816	$ 470.40
	50-59	2.4131	$ 603.28
	60+	3.1904	$ 797.60
Parent & Children			
	Under 30	2.3134	$ 578.35
	30-39	2.6261	$ 656.53
	40-49	2.7598	$ 689.95
	50-59	3.3309	$ 832.73
	60+	4.0683	$1017.08
Family			
	Under 30	2.6762	$ 669.05
	30-39	3.5248	$ 881.20
	40-49	4.1543	$1038.58
	50-59	4.6684	$1167.10
	60+	5.7874	$1446.85

These are derived from the demographic factors—the CRC factors—as discussed earlier in this volume. This is simply another application of these factors, with the sexes combined to produce "unisex" rates.

For large groups, the age/sex cost factors produce an index number which reflects the group's expected level of cost—as the weighted average of all the employees or enrollees. Here the same factors are used to produce a table, one which indicates appropriate rates by age and by contract type.

In general, rates for comprehensive plans, adjusted by age, will follow a different pattern than those for major-medical type indemnity coverages. The latter often offer limited preventive services and maternity services. That, and the effects of the deductibles and copays, produce a "grid" of rates that is different from those for an HMO.

If there are significant variations in the pattern of competitive rates, it is possible to re-allocate rates to conform. This involves some risk, because the re-allocation depends on assumptions as to the distribution of membership. Such assumptions can be guided by the knowledge of experienced actuaries. This is worth doing as there can be more risk—certainly to be avoided—in offering "non-conforming" rates in the same group market.

—#—

Small group rates, in the recent past, have been the subject of significant abuse. The overall pattern has been for carriers to apply stringent underwriting criteria, offering very low rates to "clean" groups: those known not to have any employees or dependents with serious illnesses. With the passage of time it would be assumed that the effect of such selection would wear off, with the result that rates would be increased—rapidly.

This is called "Durational Rating", and it simply involves an assumption that, starting from "clean" status, the health of the group will deteriorate, and costs will increase. The resulting rates are sometimes referred to as "select and ultimate": they would be competitive so long as the group was considered "select", with lower-than-average experience. But the "ultimate" rates, those applying to an average group, would be extremely high.

"Rate Banding" is the name applied to another small group rating practice. Here, the small group business of a carrier would be divided into segments, in accordance with the loss ratios experienced, and the carriers rate increase would be varied, so that the segment with the lowest loss ratio would get the smallest increase, that with the highest loss ratio would get the greatest increase. Here is a simplified example.

% of Small Group Business	Loss Ratio	Rate Increase
33.3%	Under 40%	5%
33.3	40-80%	15
33.4	Over 80%	30
100.0%		16.7%

The object of such stratagems was to drive out the more costly groups. Carriers played a version of "musical chairs" in which, by design, their covered groups would be winnowed down, with only the most favorable remaining.

All others would be forced to seek new coverage.

Some carriers responded to this by offering annual underwriting: if a group could show, through health questionnaires (and its claims record) that it was "clean", it would be rated as a new group.

But no group stays "clean" for long, and employers tend to value their employees, even if they get sick: they want to maintain coverage. Employers complained, and the result was a series of Small Group Acts, adopted by States in the 1990s.

These are particular to each State, and an exploration of their details could fill a volume.

The main point is that the laws limit the extent to which carriers can change or modify rates. The modifications do not have to be justified: they can be arbitrary, so long as they are uniformly applied, and the resulting rates do not exceed prescribed limits.

There are two ways in which changes are limited. The first limits the extent to which rates can be changed to recognize various attributes: health status, industry type, group size, gender, and age. Ohio, for example, allows up to a 35% variation for health status, and 35% for industry type. Connecticut will not allow variations for health status, but will allow variations for industry type (to 50%) and group size (to 25%). Massachusetts will not allow gender to be a factor in small group rates, but Ohio and Connecticut will.

The second major way in which Small Group rates are restricted is in the extent of year-to-year charge permitted for a group. A carrier is allowed to establish rate "bands", reflecting anticipated or actual experience, with the stipulations that: (1) The difference in rates—band to band—cannot exceed 15%; and (2) No group can advance by more than one band each year. The bottom line is that, for a policyholder, a rate adjustment—in addition to the general trend—cannot exceed 15%.

In sum, arbitrary changes in rates are still allowed. But they must be gradual.

It follows that in the small group market, a health plan can distinguish itself with stable rating practices.

RATING AND UNDERWRITING FOR HEALTH PLANS

PART IX

UNDERWRITING

A. THE UNDERWRITING FUNCTION

B. ORGANIZATIONAL & STAFFING CONSIDERATIONS

C. UNDERWRITING RULES

D. OBSERVATIONS ON SMALL GROUP UNDERWRITING

E. HEALTH STATEMENTS & QUESTIONNAIRES

F. OBSERVATIONS ON NON-GROUP UNDERWRITING

A. THE UNDERWRITING FUNCTION

An underwriter, in an insurance organization, has a job which can be described in terms of:

- Accepting or rejecting risks (accounts, subscriber groups);
- Arranging conditions for the acceptance of these;
- Applying appropriate rates.

This implies a decision-making function.

The word "underwriter" can also be understood in historic and literal terms: the person who *signs* on behalf of the organization, or binds it in a transaction or deal.

An underwriter in a health care organization has the same core functions as one in a casualty insurance company. But the subject matter—the nature of the risks—is different. One distinction is that a significant part of health care cost can be viewed as routine, and, on a year-to-year basis, predictable. Also, for groups, multiple insured "lives" are involved: there is pooling and hence a degree of year-to-year stability within each group. By contrast, casualty insurance is concerned with relatively infrequent occurrences: house fires, floods, car accidents, marine disasters, etc.

The underwriter in any insurance organization is the focal point of key transactions. But it is the job, not so much the individual, that occupies center stage.

An underwriter properly operates within significant constraints. These include:

- Rates, and rules for their applications, which are set forth in the organization's rate filings, which must be followed;

- Underwriting rules which guide and govern decisions in most situations;
- Precedents which must be observed in dealing equitably with covered groups.

Most underwriters occupy staff positions. They are not directly part of the organizational "chain of command". As such, they usually exercise delegated authority; the decisions they make are on behalf of the organization, as represented by the officer to whom the underwriter reports.

The underwriting process, and the decisions that are made, have to be informed by knowledge of the financial position, and underwriting capacity, of the health plan. Some plans, relatively well-capitalized, will aim for growth and in the process make "aggressive" decisions on underwriting, accepting risks which might otherwise be passed up. Other plans, wishing to conserve capital and/or to be sure of showing favorable results, will tend to be more cautious. In any event, the risk capacity of the organization is part of the information with which an underwriter must work. An underwriter then is *not* properly described as a risk-taker. Rather, the underwriter deals with risk, on behalf of the organization.

The first part of the underwriting process is *acquiring and organizing data and information*:

- about each prospective group, and each renewal account;
- about the competitive market.

A second broad set of functions involves *analysis and application of data*. For example, demographic data on a new group has to be applied to the rate factors of the health plan, so as to determine the impact of demographics on the premium rates. For renewal groups, experience data must be obtained, and, in turn, that must be applied to the plan's experience rating formula in order to indicate the appropriate level of premiums. For small groups the information obtained about the characteristics of covered employees has to be applied in a spreadsheet to build rates.

There are relatively few clear "yes/no" decisions in the underwriting process. So, a third set of functions might be characterized as *considering and applying options or conditions*. For example:

- Will the health plan be offered as a dual choice, with another plan?
- Will it be part of a multiple choice offering? Or will it be the sole carrier?
- What will the employer contribute?
- What are acceptable levels of employee contributions?

- What is the minimum level of employee participation: what percentage of eligible employees must be enrolled?
- Should a different benefit plan be offered to a subscriber group?
- How are the rates to be presented: on a 2-tier basis, 3-tier, 4-tier, 5-tier?

The main focus of such conditions is avoiding adverse selection. As discussed elsewhere in this volume, a plan's standard rates are generally matched to situations which present "normal" or typical morbidity. An employer's decisions about alternate benefit offerings, and contribution levels, can have an impact on selection. This is subject to common-sense analysis: given these choices, what can people *be expected* to do? Common sense, for experienced underwriters, is improved upon or confirmed by observations of similar situations.

The fourth broad set of functions involves *internal communications*, among the health plan's staff. If an underwriter is to function effectively within an organization, the job has to be carried out in a way that is perceived to be fair and reasonable, with the results understood by all concerned. Part of this process goes back to the first set of duties, i.e. acquiring information. When the initial information has been acquired, and analyzed, and when underwriting conditions have been considered, rates and conditions can be presented for discussion within the organization (and, under appropriate circumstances, for approval by an officer of the company). In other words, an underwriter should be able to communicate, internally, what information was available, what facts were considered, and what actions and rates are recommended. In the process, additional information may come to light, setting in motion a re-analysis.

Finally, a fifth set of functions concerns *external communications*. These mainly have to do with the explanations that will be given by the health plan in connection with proposed rates and underwriting conditions. Sometimes underwriters are asked to communicate with clients directly, but this is rare and should not be encouraged: it readily leads to situations in which the underwriter can be cast in the role of the "bad guy". For the most part, this is the point where the underwriter's function connects with that of the sales or marketing staff: these specialists are called upon to communicate with the client or account. An underwriter's main job is to be sure that the facts are clear, that the people charged with representing the plan are adequately informed, so that they, in turn, can present and discuss rates and underwriting matters.

—#—

This outline of functions is meant to emphasize that underwriting, in almost all cases, should be conducted "by the book": rates must reflect the rate filings, and precedents must be observed.

The underwriting job is important, even crucial to an organization. Bad underwriting can ruin an organization. The results of bad underwriting include:

- Inappropriate rates (too low to cover expenses, or too high to attract enrollment);
- Risks inappropriate for the organization—essentially those presenting a risk of cost fluctuation beyond the organization's capital resources and underwriting capacity;
- Inappropriate positioning in the market, generally—or in specific groups—so as to attract or encourage "adverse selection".

These considerations are such as to call for the attention of—and regular input from—the top officers of a corporation: those who understand its financial position and risk capacity.

B. ORGANIZATIONAL CONSIDERATIONS

In a smaller organization, it is usual for the Chief Operating Officer or the Chief Financial Officer to hold the decision-making role with respect to underwriting matters. The daily work involved may be assigned to underwriting analysts or technicians. In larger organizations, a senior member of the staff may hold the position of "Underwriter" or there can be an underwriting department, with a chief underwriter and a number of others.

Appropriate titles can be important. In smaller organizations, where the COO or CFO serves, effectively, as the underwriter, it is generally appropriate to recognize backup staff with accurate titles such as "underwriting assistant" or "underwriting analyst" or "underwriting technician". The term "underwriter", when applied to a job, implies familiarity with a fairly broad scope of technical knowledge, decision-making authority within the scope of the job, and a level in the organization involving regular interaction with the company's top officers. Someone who essentially serves as a technician or analyst should *not* be described as an underwriter: just as a sergeant should not be addressed as a captain or a major.

In organizational terms, underwriting is ordinarily considered a "staff" function, a step outside of the decision-making line of authority or the governance structure. While an underwriter exercises decision-making authority, this usually is delegated (unless the underwriter is as described earlier, an officer of a smaller health plan). It derives from the authority inherent in the position of the officer to whom the underwriter reports. This could be the President, CEO, Chief Operating Officer, or Chief Financial Officer. That is, the underwriter works with, and within, the authority granted by his or her boss.

Health plan underwriters are expected—within the scope of their jobs—to use facts to come to determinations or decisions. In that sense, an underwriter is expected to be independent, to come to his/her own conclusions. These are properly characterized as determinations: based on objective facts. (Opinions, based on instinct, are another matter.)

In some cases, some underwriting tasks are handled by members of the marketing or sales staffs, under the authority, for example, of the Vice President for Sales and Marketing. This can be appropriate *if* the job is that of a technician, limited to the mechanical aspect of developing rate quotes. Otherwise a job with broader scope—that of an underwriter—can be regarded as involving a conflict of interest. The main underwriting functions are to assure that the organization will not be saddled with excessive or inappropriate risks, and to assure that rates are adequate. Pursuing these goals inevitably involve taking positions contrary to that of the marketing staff. Combining both sets of goals invites dysfunction, or at least a serious headache.

It is almost axiomatic that there will be tension between the sales staff—bent on getting new enrollees and keeping customers happy—and an underwriter, who is mainly charged with protecting the financial interests of the organization.

In fact, the job of the underwriter should involve controversy: dealing regularly with issues involving premium rates and enrollment. This can be viewed as normal, usual and healthy. If the essential conflict or tension is acknowledged and institutionalized, the marketing staff is free to advocate for the enrollment of any interested group, and for the lowest rates possible, while the underwriter, or underwriting department, acts as counterweight and looks to the suitability of the risks, and the adequacy of rates. In healthy organizations, people can "fight" constantly: in the sense of representing different points of view. But they have to "fight fair".

This can lead to very productive working relationships. For example, marketers can learn what information the underwriter needs and make sure it is presented up front. Underwriters can learn to understand the challenges faced by marketers, and options—in approaching subscriber groups—can be hashed out in advance.

From an organizational perspective, it is imperative to recognize and accommodate differing viewpoints or sets of goals, allowing the people involved the opportunity to achieve their own balance in their working relationships. Different positions can be clearly understood as stemming from different jobs, and should not result in real animosity.

This goal can be furthered by management, through, first, making clear the purposes of the organization; second, through defining the jobs expected to be done by the underwriters and the sales staff; and third, by being available to exercise decision-making authority, in situations which are not routine and which cannot be resolved by staff. The latter point should be especially emphasized. If staff members are expected to argue or disagree, someone has to be available to serve as a tie-breaker.

Also, when underwriters are expected to live by the rules, someone has to be available to step in to deal with extraordinary situations: those not contemplated by the rules. There *are* occasions in which a CEO may, for good reason, decide to bet his job, and/or the future of the health plan, on a decision which may be viewed as instinctive (or, to some, just plain nuts.) In such cases, the job of the underwriter is to assist and provide information. It is never the job of the underwriter to "go by his gut": the boss gets to do that.

C. UNDERWRITING RULES

Underwriting rules are mainly relevant for smaller and mid-sized groups. For larger groups—say 500 employees and up—most health plans do not usually raise the question of whether to offer coverage, or present substantial conditions for enrollment. For such larger groups, it is generally considered that the rigors of full time employment—mainly keeping regular hours—is an effective "screen", eliminating most people with functional impairments. Also, for larger groups, experience, after the first year or so of coverage, will dictate the level of charges. So, for big groups, the decisions that need to be made are not likely to concern the conditions of coverage. Instead the main job is getting the initial rate right.

But—for most of its business—every insuring organization must have underwriting policies and rules to help assure that it will not be saddled with excessive or inappropriate risks. This is a defensive posture, and a necessary one.

The rules should be written, and clear.

And each set of rules, ideally, is specific to a particular plan: its *own* rules. "Underwriting rules" can be copied or passed along from one organization to another, without much thought as to applicability and relevance. Such rules, having been imported and being poorly understood, are usually not fully observed: they can be seen as irrelevant . . . because they are!

Each health plan should go through a process of internalizing its underwriting rules.

There are various ways to do this: we advocate a process of developing "home-grown" rules—focused on the real situation faced by the health plan.

Such rules are really answers to some key questions. These concern:

(1) Marketing Targets and Appeals;
(2) Organization and Management;
(3) Group Qualification;

(4) Alternate Coverages—conditions for participation in multiple choice situations;
(5) Participation Requirements;
(6) Employment Verification;
(7) Cost Differentials or Out-of-Pocket Expense;
(8) Choice of Benefit Plan.

Separate, and different, rules can apply to larger groups and to smaller groups. On the following pages, we will review the considerations which shape the answers, and the resulting rules.

(1) *Marketing Targets and Appeals*

An important aspect of sound underwriting is market position, and the determination of the sales appeals or representations which may be made. How does the plan characterize itself? What reasons are given for encouraging enrollment? What sorts of people are addressed by marketing appeals? What advantages are claimed for enrollment in this plan?

The answers to such questions have no direct relationship to the day-to-day work of preparing rate quotes. But they are a big part of the process by which the plan attracts and retains members.

So these should be clear answers. In turn, these must be repeated in public relations and advertising, and emphasized by the plan's representatives.

Adverse selection can be a byproduct of consumer decisions when a health plan adopts the traditional appeals of group insurance, emphasizing the complete protection available, and focusing enrollment appeals on fear of the financial consequences of serious illness. Similar results can come from emphasis on affiliations with leading medical centers, etc. Health plans can seek more balanced selection through emphasizing the interests of the well, such as care in pregnancy and childbirth, routine pediatric care, prompt attention to athletic injuries, etc.

The long-term aim, of course, is simply to attract (and retain) groups with *average* health care needs, appropriate to the rates being charged. Enrollment will occur for many reasons, and the plan's self-characterization or description—the headlines in its ads—will tend to diminish in importance as enrollment grows: what people think of the organization and its service ultimately takes precedence.

But it is still necessary for a health plan to keep alert to its self-description. Attributes to be emphasized need not focus directly on a quest for favorable selection, or avoidance of adverse selection. In competition for the attention of consumers, long-term advantages, particularly in member retention, can come from emphasizing the quality of care provided to members, the ways in which the organization helps members maintain health, and the sincerity of its commitments to positive health outcomes. Such messages start from the top: management has to be able to articulate why its plan should be chosen. In turn, this describes to employees and sales staffs how they can best present the plan.

(2) *Organization and Management*

Underwriting policies, as well as incentive compensation for sales, should assure that the marketing and enrollment staffs adhere to sound policies with respect to sales appeals: what is said or promised to persuade people to join. This, we believe, requires frequent and thoughtful attention. Except in the situation of phone sales (to very small accounts) people making marketing presentations simply cannot be monitored as they do their work. But their messages need to be not only persuasive, but also consistent with the purposes of the plan.

Another aspect of organization for the application of underwriting policies is the designation of a person or group to resolve questions as to the application of formal rules. (As noted earlier, there are circumstances in which a rule will be modified, interpreted, waived, or even broken.) Such a person or group must be in a position to balance enrollment objectives and market imperatives with the organizational need to avoid creating inappropriate precedents. This is not something for the underwriter to do: it is something for the top officers and, in some circumstances, the Board of Directors.

(3) *Group Qualification*

(a) *Industry*. Various rules can be made regarding the basic qualifications of eligible groups. These are often expressed in terms of lists of "desirable" and "undesirable" industries or occupations. Such lists often have an historic origin in insurance company observations of so-called "moral hazard" and/or occupational health risk and/or relative cost. Thus saloons, junkyards, etc. are often listed as "undesirable". However, these observations may not have been based on data in the first place and also may not be relevant to contemporary local reality. Rules based on such ancient lists may be considered as "red-lining" and not acceptable to state regulators.

It is most productive to focus attention on whether the employee group is a *stable* one, working regularly. Generally to be avoided are situations involving casual or short-term employment, without requirement of substantial skill and/or attachment to the employer's business. If employees are hired on a casual basis, then the group can include people who are unusually compromised in terms of health status.

A classic example may be something like a car wash establishment: one in which new employees need no knowledge other than that which they will learn in the first hour or so of work. One employee can easily be replaced with another. So such a business may be in a near-continuous process of hiring, on the basis that if one employee doesn't work out, the next one will. (With that approach, there is likely no interest in health coverage.)

Such observations need not necessarily exclude or "red-line" all businesses doing the same kind of work: some may be operated by regular long-term employees. This is true of restaurants, hotels, and other service establishments: most involve revolving-door employment, but some do not. The real characteristics of the organization should override, or supersede, a broad industry exclusion.

(b) *Financial Stability.* Employer financial stability is another consideration. Insurers generally want to avoid situations where collection problems can be anticipated.

This can lead to the regular use of credit rating services, such as Dun and Bradstreet. Such services may not complete information, but they generally have enough of it to warn of likely impending problems.

Some carriers follow a rule that a business has to be in existence for a certain length of time to qualify for coverage. In general, this can exclude many viable prospects: application of other criteria (such as a clean credit report) gets to the heart of the matter.

(c) *Workers Compensation.* Health care coverage offered as an employee benefit is intended, and priced, to cover *non-occupational* illnesses and injuries. Workers compensation coverage *must* be a requirement. If members do not have workers compensation coverage, it is possible for the health plan to become liable for the cost of treatment for occupational injuries, without intending to do so, and without charging a premium for that.

(4) *Alternate Coverages*

This underwriting question has to do with the other coverages offered by a subscriber group to each employer. Health plans generally seek to be the "exclusive" carrier for as many employers as possible. Selection is a consideration. If there can be no selection on the part of the employees, then it can't be adverse, at least within the group. Also, an "exclusive" kicks competitors out: out of sight, hopefully out of mind, and no threat. The belief, essentially, is that a health plan is in a much stronger position as the exclusive carrier.

Another point of view, which was held forth as a principle by early group practice prepayment plans, is that the employer *must* have another health insurance program: at least one other option which employees can choose. The idea here is to provide a safety valve: those dissatisfied with, or even wary of, a plan's care-management activities could go elsewhere. (Such a position, if widely adopted, would markedly reduce the extent to which people could imagine that their well-being may be threatened, and in turn would reduce demand for government regulation of health plans through "patients' rights" legislation.)

There is, in short, something to be said for the continuing involvement of another carrier. That permits the plan to, in effect, "be itself" and not attempt to meet the needs and preferences of all. By offering a choice of plans, an employer can increase the value of the benefit plan offering—the extent to which it is valued or appreciated by employees.

Where there is choice in a group it is important to understand the dynamics of how this will play out to affect employee selection of health plans. The main concern here is relative price, although other characteristics and attributes can play a part. The position to avoid, in general, is being the highest-priced carrier and/or one which has the greatest appeal to people with significant health problems.

(5) *Participation Requirements*

To avoid adverse selection, long-standing insurance industry practices require that a specified percentage of the group be enrolled, or that a minimum number of people be enrolled, before a group contract can become effective. But for small groups, 100% enrollment may be required. A minimum of, for example, 15 contracts may be required in groups employing more than 20 but less than 30 people.

Though the participation required may be important, it tends to lose meaning in small groups, where a significant portion of the work force may decline coverage, either because of existing coverage through another family member, or because of the expense. This places more emphasis on employment verification, discussed next.

(6) *Employment Verification*

The most important single aspect of underwriting, for smaller groups, is verification of actual full-time employment.

It has been observed that the rigors of regular employment effectively exclude impaired people from employment with most larger groups. But smaller groups tend to have considerable flexibility in whom they hire, the regularity of required attendance at work, etc. Accordingly, small business proprietors are in a position to do favors for family members and friends, by listing them as employees and acting as a conduit for employment-based health insurance. This includes covering people who in fact work part-time, or only work occasionally, and may include covering people who really aren't employed at all in the enterprise.

The underwriting dangers are obvious in the sense that the usual "screen"—employee fitness for regular work—is not present. In turn, this means that the rates can be inadequate: these are ordinarily based on the experience generated by full-time employees and their enrolled dependents.

The underwriting solution is generally fairly straightforward: a requirement that the employer produce, for review and inspection, payroll tax reports or a similar government-required document. These should be reviewed by the underwriter when coverage begins, and spot-checked thereafter. Another safeguard can be a requirement that the enrollment representative periodically visit the workplace and ascertain the work locations and duties of each of the employees.

(7) *Cost Differential or Out-of-Pocket Expense*

A health plan should attempt to assure that it will not be excessively high-priced in relation to other coverages available to employees. A common standard is that the differential (between the offering plan's rate and that of an alternate carrier) should not exceed 25%. More to the point, this can also be expressed in terms of relative out-of-pocket costs to employees. But rules on this subject should not be overly rigid. They have to be adapted as employers pay smaller portions of total premiums. The object, of course, is the same as for other underwriting rules: avoiding adverse selection.

(8) *Choice of Benefit Plan*

Health plan underwriting rules may also address the question of whether a low-option or a high-option coverage will be offered to a particular group. In general, the aim is to assure that, to the extent possible, the offering plan's prices (and out-of-pocket expenses to the employee) will be affordable.

Developing Rules

The observation was made that *real* underwriting rules reflect a consensus of the people in an organization, reflecting its policies. Therefore they are followed.

So, we suggest, a thoughtful process of developing real and relevant underwriting rules is very useful, if not essential. It is also, we suggest, not difficult. The "technique" is essentially to convene an appropriate forum, within the organization, to discuss a series of questions. Input from a knowledgeable consultant can be useful, but the rules should reflect the organization's own judgments and conclusions, based on its own circumstances, its understanding of the market, and related factors. A list of possible topics for such a discussion—and a resulting set of rules—follows:

Restrictions on Market
- Employer group size?
- Types of business?

Qualifications for Employer Groups
- Stability—what measures?
- Viability—what measures?

Eligibility Rules
- Minimum requirements?
- Standard rule?

Participation Requirement
- Basic Rules?
- Variations by size?
- Exceptions permitted?
- Exclusive carrier? When?

Enrollment
- When permitted?
- Handling of new hires?
- Handling of changes in dependency status?

Benefit Design
- Price considerations?
- Market comparison?
- Underwriting/risk considerations?
- State requirements?

Alternate Carriers/Competitors
- Dual choice required? Permitted?
- Multiple choice permitted?
- Comparative benefit plans?
- Comparative premiums?
- Comparative employer/employee contributions?

Underwriting History
- What information to get?
- Decisions? Rules? Guidelines?

Rate Tier Structure
- Standard?
- Adapted to group/competition: How?

Employment Test
- Minimum work requirement (hours per week)?
- Regular employment (weeks per year)?
- Proofs required?
- Enforcement?

It will be recognized that many of the answers have been suggested, though not prescribed, by observations in the preceding text.

A final observation is that in defining underwriting rules, it can be useful not to become too detailed. The object should be kept in mind, and that can be simply defined as a set of guidelines which will help the organization:

- Do business with employer groups which are reasonably stable and solvent;
- Enroll people whose health care needs conform with the experience and expectations which underlie the rates.

D. OBSERVATIONS ON SMALL GROUP UNDERWRITING

Small groups (generally under 25 employees) represent a significant market.

These are distinguished from larger groups in at least two ways.

(1) *Administration and Marketing.* Expense allocations should be adequate to sustain the costs of dealing with smaller groups. Special personnel should be devoted to these tasks: the job of marketing to smaller employers (and their employees) is different from the process of dealing with larger employers. It may consist mainly of dealing with brokers. In markets where brokers do not control small-group business, a plan's marketing to small groups should follow a regular plan, and schedule, of calls and presentations. Premium accounting and collection rules also should be specific to the small group market. These do not incorporate the flexibility which may be allowed in dealings with larger groups.

(2) *Underwriting.* Special attention is needed, including consideration of the following.

    (a) *Employment Verification.* As discussed in the preceding section, employment verification is the key element in underwriting for small groups. As noted, it is easy for many small groups to harbor or host, as occasional or "phantom" employees, people whose health status will not permit regular full-time work. While coverage of such persons is a public policy issue, commercially—competitive rates are the goal of a health plan. Accordingly, *enforcement of an* "*actively at work*" *requirement is the single most important matter to be addressed in small group underwriting.*

Active surveillance is appropriate. In turn, there are two simple indicators of whether a claimed employee is actually at work: a) Are payroll taxes paid for this employee? And b) Is there a place for this employee at the work site? (If home-based or "in-the-field" employment is claimed, are the conditions for this believable, realistic?)

(b) *Qualification of Employers.* Policies and guidelines for the small group market concern the acceptance/rejection of employers which are judged to reflect a more-than-usual risk of bankruptcy, termination of employment, or the enrollment of adverse risks. As noted earlier, there are traditional lists of the kinds of business to avoid: generally the underlying trend is to steer clear of those characterized by low-skill, short-term employment and businesses with low odds of permanence. Those thought of as hazardous are also generally avoided (even though non-occupational coverage is offered, and work hazards must be covered by workers' compensation). But each health plan should consider its own objectives and rules in this regard. Since only non-occupational coverage is offered, does it really matter that the work might be considered hazardous? If employment in a particular restaurant is stable, does it matter that, in general, restaurants usually don't have many long-term employees?

(c) *Nature of the Competition.* In some markets, the main sources of coverage for small employers are indemnity insurance companies, which generally employ very strict underwriting guidelines, charge "what the market will bear," and offer limited coverage. But this isn't universally true: Blue Cross/Blue Shield plans in some locations, and some HMOs, offer comprehensive coverage at reasonable prices. It is necessary to be sure that a relevant competitive product is offered, with an appropriate rate structure, and at an appropriate price.

(d) *Market Segmentation.* The small group market in an area may be divided into categories, mainly based on size. One possible result is the identification of categories which will be enrolled using only the restrictions and standards appropriate to non-group coverage. Other distinctions may be developed: possibly making separate categories of medium-sized (25-50 employees), small (10-24 employees) and very small (3-9) groups. *Note*: Some experts conclude that, below some threshold—10-15 employees, a group is not really a group but is an aggregation of individuals.

(e) *Plans of Benefits.* Coverages offered in the small group market can be less comprehensive than those usually provided according to HMO standards or rules. A major reason for this is that the health insurance contributions of smaller employers are often meager, and so is the coverage offered. A health plan with comprehensive coverage and relatively high premium costs stands in strong danger of adverse selection, if it seeks to compete in a market dominated by "thin" coverage.

(f) *Health Questionnaires.* Many insurers in the small group market use health questionnaires to ascertain if a group qualifies for coverage: essentially these are intended to identify people with current health care needs. Ordinarily the underwriting decisions arising from such a review involve the rejection or acceptance of the entire group, or the assignment of a small group to a rate band. Health questionnaires are not generally permitted to be used in rejecting individuals for coverage, or for setting special rates, by persons based on health risk.

(g) *Participation Requirements.* In the small group market, it is usual to enroll the entire group, without the possibility of dual choice. Similarly, an underwriting requirement to enroll a certain portion of the group is usual and appropriate: for example, a group will not be enrolled unless at least 75% or 67% of eligible employees join the plan. Such a requirement helps to spread the risk and to guard against adverse selection.

(h) *Pre-Existing Conditions.* Pre-existing condition clauses, once common, have generally been banished by legislation. Before imposing any such requirement, it is necessary to check whether it is permissible.

If enrollment is limited to those *without* current health problems, the enrolled group is considered "select" and is likely to enjoy favorable experience (to the extent of about a 10%—20% reduction in costs, depending on the stringency of the risk-selection process) for about two or three years after enrollment. Following this, the phenomenon known as "regression to the mean" can be expected: that is, the effect of selection wears off, and the group is progressively more likely to exhibit typical needs and costs.

(i) *Rates Specific to the Risk.* The simplicity of rate structures for large groups is mainly in response to custom and to employer preference. That is, larger employers have become accustomed to two-tier rates, three-tier rates, or composite rates. But smaller employers are more flexible. Rates particular to the risks are advisable:

- five-tier rate structures (single, parent/child, parent/children, couple, family);
- possible add-ons for large families (more than three children);
- rate-book pricing, i.e. different rates by age group.

The latter involves the use of a schedule of rates which are specific for each contract type and for each subscriber age classification. Thus an employer might be billed in accordance with a matrix of rates (5 contract types, 7 to 11 age bands—or a total of 35 to 55 separate rates). The health plan's billing would take the form of a listing of covered employees, with a rate for each, with space on the remittance form for the employer list additions and deletions. Thus the aggregate rate accommodates to changes in the enrolled work force.

E. HEALTH STATEMENTS AND QUESTIONNAIRES

In small groups, prospective enrollees are usually asked to fill out a health questionnaire.

The completed questionnaires are then evaluated, for two essential purposes: (a) to decide whether or not to accept the group; and (b) to assign the group to the appropriate band (reflecting anticipated relative cost) if rate bands are part of the rating format.

Most managed care plans use standard questionnaires which generally address the following:

(1) Specified diseases. Does any prospective enrollee currently have any of a list of diseases or conditions? These can include, for example, heart disease, cancer, diabetes, psychosis/psychoneurosis, drug/alcohol dependency, emphysema, coronary artery disease, acquired immune deficiency syndrome (AIDS), epilepsy, high blood pressure, kidney disease.
(2) Who has been hospitalized recently? In the last 12 months? What for?
(3) Who is taking prescription medications for a chronic condition? Which drugs, which conditions?

A plan's Medical Director can be helpful in formulating a policy for review of these medical questionnaires. They should not be subjectively reviewed; instead it is appropriate to devise a point system, so as to facilitate the development of an objective score. Such a system can be developed from a review of claims records for a span of time: identifying the most costly conditions.

Health questionnaires are widely used in the initial assessment of small groups. But the importance of these should not be over-emphasized: the main thing accomplished by the use of such questionnaires is to alert a plan to expensive, chronic conditions affecting dependents of enrollees in new groups. Once a group is accepted for coverage, medical underwriting falls by the wayside: in most jurisdictions, questionnaires can only be required of those who enroll late; that is, employees who do not take up coverage when they are first eligible. The most important underwriting condition, in all events, is the "actively at work" requirement.

F. OBSERVATIONS ON NON-GROUP UNDERWRITING

Non-group coverage presents special underwriting hazards and challenges, but can represent a viable line of business.

People eligible for non-group coverage are generally in population groups with more-than-usual health care risks. This does not mean that *all* non-group enrollees inherently carry extraordinary risk: but many high-risk people *can* be included.

Recognizing the hazards, special attention needs to be devoted to considerations of benefit design, pricing, underwriting, marketing, and administration affecting non-group business.

Caution and care are strongly suggested. The prospects for significant loss are readily at hand, and a mis-step can be expensive. On the other hand, non-group coverage *need not* be a money-losing proposition: it *can* be viable.

To help assure that non-group coverage is viable, the following practical matters should be considered.

(1) *Recognize classifications of potential enrollees.* Non-group coverage (apart from Medicare) mainly affects three categories of people:

   (a) employed people who do not fall in the group category, such as independent professionals, people who work as independent contractors, etc.;
   (b) People who join during open-enrollment periods, who may or may not be employed, or whose part-time employment is too limited to qualify for group coverage;
   (c) People who have left employment and who convert group coverage to non-group.

Each category differs from the other in terms of risk, including employment status, and the likelihood of adverse selection.

The importance of conversion coverage as such is lessened by the Consolidated Omnibus Reconciliation Act of 1985 (COBRA). This requires employers of more than 24 employees to make group coverage available for at least 18 months in case of termination of employment, and for 36 months for certain dependents who lose eligibility. Since such COBRA-eligible people are carried as eligible members of groups, it is not usually practical to treat them as a separate class or category. It is clear, however, that the remaining conversions include people who have been unemployed for longer times.

(2) *Use health statements.* These have historically been used for new non-group enrollments (not for conversions):

   (a) To assign people to coverage and/or rating classes;
   (b) To enforce a waiting period for coverage of pre-existing conditions.

   There are at least two concerns about using health statements, however. The first is whether this is currently permitted in the jurisdiction. The second is administrative feasibility: what medical rules will be applied? Are they clear and defensible?

(3) *Limit the coverage offered.* This serves at least two purposes:

   (a) It reduces the risk exposure of the health plan;
   (b) It makes the coverage more affordable, and hence lessens the risk of adverse selection.

(4) *Vary the rates by category.* Three sub-parts of the non-group "market" were noted (in No. 1 above). Each, potentially, could have a different rate, based on observed experience in each category, and on prospective determinants of utilization. Also, there are at least two objective bases for rate distinctions within non-group classifications:

   (a) It has been observed that, on average, unemployed non-group subscribers have significantly worse experience than those who are employed: this can be a basis for a distinction within a CRC system, or the basis for an experience-based differential.
   (b) Age/sex rating is readily possible, and can equalize the risk to the

HMO arising from a disproportionate number of older people. A rate-book approach, as discussed in connection with small group enrollment, is a practical necessity, since this is the way rates of most competing carriers are structured.

(5) *Charge adequately for administrative expenses.* The expenses of billing and the collection losses on non-group coverage are much higher than for group coverage.

(6) *Note the market environment.* In different markets, health plans are more or less vulnerable to adverse selection in non-group enrollment. HMOs in areas of especially high unemployment might encounter conversions among relatively young people, for example, reflecting more on the absence of job opportunities than on health impairments. Attention to such environmental factors helps to make the response to non-group underwriting more focused and relevant to the situation.

(7) *Use open-enrollment periods.* The use of time-limited open-enrollment periods has proved to be very effective in limiting adverse selection. It is considered reasonable to assume that if people can get health care coverage whenever they need it, they will tend to defer enrollment until the need for care is at hand, or at least in their minds. On the other hand, an enrollment "drive," with the opportunity for enrollment limited to a certain period of time, is likely to attract a balanced population—mostly people who simply think it is a good idea to be covered.

PART X

END NOTES

END NOTES

Underwriting and rate-setting are crucial for any health plan: success obviously depends upon charging appropriate prices, and on matching rates to the risks. Mistakes and surprises are to be avoided.

The amounts of money involved in health care coverage are huge, margins for carriers are small, competition is intense, and minor mistakes can set the stage for financial disaster. No health plan can stand the unwelcome financial surprises which can result from unsophisticated underwriting or casual approaches to rate-setting.

Methodical, thoughtful, careful approaches are in order.

The essence of sophistication in rate-setting is not cleverness or cunning, nor is it "the art of the deal." Instead, it is the systematic application of rational methods. First, this means that each health plan must define its rating approaches and build a rating structure. The rating process, in turn, requires the collection, analysis, and use of facts, and consistency in the application of rules.

These rules are not, by and large, externally imposed. Instead, these are devised by the health plans themselves, based on their understanding of their own interests.

Managed care programs have unique features. They can learn from group insurance practices, but the templates and practices of "traditional" carriers do not fully apply to managed care programs. Further, since each health plan is unique, no universal methods can apply: each plan needs structures for rating and underwriting to suit its own circumstances—its own risk arrangements, its risk capacity, its market, and its regulatory environment.

All health care prepayment organizations must, like all risk-taking carriers, pay attention to underwriting. Underwriting requirements cannot—as a practical matter—be used to select only the best risks. Instead the purpose of underwriting rules, carefully developed and fairly applied, is to assure each carrier that the risks it accepts will be appropriate for its risk capacity, and consistent with the rates it charges. Each organization will approach underwriting in its own way, with its own rules. These rules must be thought out: they must fit the situation.

The health plan "market" is dynamic. We anticipate that plans will increasingly recognize the costs of their assuming risk, and will charge for it. Employers, in turn, will refine their view of the market, seeking services and products which meet their interests. The process of adaptation is ongoing.

An aim of this volume is to describe the elements of a framework around which appropriate and workable rating and risk structures can be built.

In the development and application of regular rules and practices, it is important to understand why they exist, and the available options. We hope that this volume will help health plans in using knowledgeable approaches to rate-setting and underwriting.